Flip THE Switch

ALSO BY JIM KARAS

THE BUSINESS PLAN FOR THE BODY

Flip THE Switch

DISCOVER THE WEIGHT-LOSS SOLUTION AND
THE SECRET TO GETTING STARTED

JIM KARAS

HARMONY BOOKS • NEW YORK

This book proposes a program of physical exercise and dietary recommendations for the reader to follow. However, before starting this or any other exercise program or diet regimen, you should consult your physician.

Published by Harmony Books, New York, New York
Member of the Crown Publishing Group, a division of Random House, Inc.
www.randomhouse.com

HARMONY BOOKS is a registered trademark and the Harmony Books colophon is a trademark of Random House, Inc.

Printed in the United States of America

DESIGN BY ELINA D. NUDELMAN

PHOTOGRAPHS BY BETH BISCHOFF

LINE ART ILLUSTRATIONS BY JACKIE AHER

Library of Congress Cataloging-in-Publication Data

Karas, Jim.
    Flip the switch: discover the weight-loss solution and the secret to getting started / Jim Karas.— 1st ed.
    Includes bibliographical references and index.
    1. Weight loss—Psychological aspects—Popular works.   I. Title.
    RM222.2 .K3373 2002
    613.7—dc21   2002032884

ISBN 1-4000-45959

10 9 8 7 6 5 4 3 2 1

First Edition

To Olivia and Evan, you're the best

Acknowledgments

First I would like to thank my agent, Amanda (Binky) Urban at ICM, and my publicist, Sandy Mendelson of Hilsinger/Mendelson. They don't know this, but I call them my "A" team girls, since they are smart, fast, funny, and totally results oriented. Plus, they have husbands, careers, and kids and find time to exercise and eat a healthy diet. You'll appreciate this point more when you read the book.

Next I would like to thank my New York contingency, Diane, Sherrie, Phyllis, Peggy, Marie, Maria, Loretto, Ellen, Dick, Shelley, and David who make working in New York a blast. A special thanks to Marie Brenner for sharing her personal history (check it out in Chapter 9) with me and with all of you.

I also want to single out Diane Sawyer. When you see her on television, she is smart, charming, beautiful, and witty. When I see her to work out, she is exactly the same minus the high heels. She puts up with my (what I think are funny) motivational e-mails and voice-mail messages, continues to be the "Jim Karas Poster Child for Weight Loss," and has done so many wonderful things for me that they are too many to list. Thanks, Diane, I'm so glad you didn't deck me the first time we met when I told you that you were twenty-five pounds overweight!

I have to thank two people I call my "sisters," Patti Salvagio (my model in the pictures in Chapter 8) and Cynthia Costas Cohen. I never had a sister, but both of you constantly give me such love and support, even when I act up, as little brothers do sometimes. We all believe in something we call "the power," which is basically a belief that you can accomplish whatever you want if you set your mind to it. I hope we never lose it and never lose our bond.

Some of us are lucky enough to have a best friend; I have one in Bob Lang. As he did with my first book, *The Business Plan for the Body,* he helped me craft this book's proposal and gave ongoing advice about form and shape. He also helped me (along with my terrific business manager, Jeff Connell) to repair the numerous computers that just don't seem to like my style. I believe banging on a mouse motivates it to perform. They have advised me otherwise.

To my wife, Ellen, who is holding up well given that she is working again, taking care of two active kids, and dealing with an often absent husband. Just know you're doing a great job, and thanks for letting me tell some of your more "personal" issues with weight loss.

Finally to my kids, Olivia and Evan. I always say that my life has never been the same since the day Olivia popped on the scene. I feel such an overwhelming love for her. Then, it happened all over again with Evan. I talk so much about all of our early programming in this book. I hope, as your parent, that I am giving you the right foundation to be happy, healthy, productive, well-adjusted adults. (Okay, to be fair, I'll settle for medium happy, very healthy, semi-productive, and moderately well-adjusted adults. Why put pressure on you to be perfect?) You make just about everything fun and have made my life complete. I hope that years from now, when you read this book as adults, you will smile and know that, as most parents do, I only wanted the best for you.

Contents

Part III: Living Flipped

Introduction

"Though no one can go back and make a brand-new start, anyone can start from now and make a brand-new ending." I have always loved this quote. Whenever I am feeling overwhelmed I stop and, though I realize that there is nothing I can do to erase the past, I tell myself that I can, from this point forward, lay the groundwork for the future. You, too, can do the same.

Several years ago, a dietitian named Anne Fletcher conducted a survey of 160 individuals who successfully met their weight-loss goals. What separated the losers from the "losers" was referred to as the proverbial "flip of the switch" in which the desire to lose weight finally became more important than the desire to overeat and not to exercise. That's what I am urging you to do once and for all, *decide that your desire to succeed at weight loss is greater than your desire to fail.* Then take that desire and turn it into a reality. I know you can do it. Just "flip the switch."

Millions of Americans possess the desire to lose weight, yet so few succeed. Why? The decision to translate that desire into action and lose weight must come from *within* an individual. A spouse or partner can't make you do it, a parent can't make you do it, a friend can't make you do it. Only you can make that decision to lose weight. If you review most of the successes in your life, they occurred because you established a clear goal, then determined a path to achieve that goal. More important, you believed that the goal you *chose* could and would be *achieved.* The same happens with weight loss. Decide that once and for all you can win at weight loss, then transform that desire into a reality.

How do you move to the point where the desire to succeed is greater than the desire to fail? In other words, how

> "ONLY I CAN CHANGE MY LIFE. NO ONE CAN DO IT FOR ME."
> —Carol Burnett

do you reach what I call "the flipping point"? In my first book, *The Business Plan for the Body*, I gave readers a comprehensive action plan for success at weight loss based upon the structured components of a classic American business plan. What surprised me was not the number of sales, but the number of readers who e-mailed, wrote, or faxed me letters stating that they loved the concepts outlined in the book but just couldn't find a way to emotionally commit themselves to get started at weight loss. So, that is the goal of this book. I want to give you the tools to examine each of the potential obstacles that have kept you from flipping and help you to eliminate them one by one or at least assist you in managing them to your advantage.

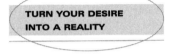

TURN YOUR DESIRE
INTO A REALITY

Are You Ready to Flip?

Most weight-loss books fail because they try to impose or apply a quick, easy solution to a highly complex problem. So many times, weight-loss books give you an eating and/or exercise program, assuming that you are ready to go and have already mentally committed to losing weight. Unfortunately, these books often are not addressing the powerful emotional issues that surround weight loss. Throughout this book, we will continually return to the "core issues" in your life: your childhood, your feelings about your body, your relationship to family, food, and physical activity. We'll analyze the role they've played as factors in your struggle to flip. You probably will be surprised to see how many of these elements, some of which may reside in your subconscious, have conspired to sabotage your will to flip. By closely examining these factors and avoiding a Band-Aid solution, such as a quick-fix diet or an excessive exercise program, we will rebuild your inner core and subsequently approach your weight-loss strategy on a firmer emotional foundation.

Certain pages of this book are designed in an interactive workbook format. I will ask you to complete specific exercises and record your responses to various questions in the space provided. These exercises are meant to provoke thought and provide you with a written journal as you connect with your inner core and move through the flipping process. Consequently, you will be producing a written record of your journey. That way, whenever you feel you need encouragement or support, you can leaf through the book and review all the thoughts, emotions, and exercises that led you to your decision to flip.

I Flipped, So Can You

Many years ago I flipped the switch. Unlike most in the weight-loss field who may never have had to deal with losing weight, I have had to deal with it each and every day. And believe me, I don't want to flip the switch off again. One of my reasons for writing this book is to share with you my own struggle, and the struggle of thousands of individuals whom I have coached over the years to success. Of course, along the way there have been some failures. But you know what? We learn from those failures (I definitely did) and they can help us avoid similar mistakes in our own strategy. The individuals who failed started this journey, but at some point along the way decided to turn back. You are not going to turn back. I will guarantee you don't get caught in the same traps and thus lose the opportunity to stay flipped for life.

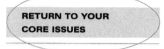

RETURN TO YOUR
CORE ISSUES

To gain additional information, I've reviewed research conducted by psychologists and psychiatrists in the field of weight loss. This research has provided me with a deeper and more comprehensive understanding of the highly emotional complexity surrounding the decision to lose weight, stay on course, and succeed at living flipped for life.

How to Use This Book

We begin our examination in Part 1, "It Can Happen to You." In the first chapter, "Believe in the Flip," I explain to you that to achieve success at weight loss, you must first believe in your ability to do so. Throughout this book, you are asked to complete a series of written exercises that examine past and present feelings about your body, body weight, and body image. In Chapter 2, "Visualize the Flip," I urge you to use the powerful tool of visualization to create a mental picture of a thinner, healthier, more attractive you. In other words, visualize your goal. Believing in yourself and visualizing the outcome of that belief will pave the way to successful weight loss.

In Part 2, "What's Kept *You* from Flipping?," I draw from my fifteen years of experience as a weight-loss consultant. I have heard all the excuses, rationales, alibis, and objections repeated hundreds, if not thousands, of times. I will admit that some of them do possess a degree of validity. Most of them, however, simply require intelligent management to ensure that as you move through this process of flipping, no one barrier thwarts your desire and ability to succeed. From Chapter 3, "'I Don't Have the Time,'" through Chapter 10, "'It's Just Too Late,'" we discuss each of these issues and together devise an action plan to overcome those beliefs, situations, or circumstances that appear to be in your way. After reading Chapters 1 and 2, you may skip directly to the barrier that you feel most applies to you, though for most individuals, the book is designed to build on themes in the order they have been presented. Taking action is the central theme of Part 2.

Here's an example. If you frequently say you don't have time in your present schedule to fit in exercise and healthy eating habits, I will show you in Chapter 3, "'I Don't Have the Time,'" how you can carve out the time to exercise and make wiser food choices. Keep in mind, there are lots of people in this world who are busier than you who find the time to do it—and so can you. You will benefit, your family will benefit, your friends will benefit, and your workplace/ employer will benefit. There's no question that it's a win-win endeavor. Similarly, in Chapter 8, "'I Hate to Exercise,'" I will explain to you the numerous benefits of exercise with regard to not only weight loss but improved posture, confidence, and the ability to live a long, pain-free, independent life. I know you have previously heard discussions of these benefits, but I will demonstrate how they can apply specifically to you and your current environment. I will show you how to exercise effectively in a limited amount of time. Note that phrase: "limited amount of time." Please don't think I am one of those weight-loss experts who espouses the benefits of two hours of exercise each and every day. That in my opinion is not only unrealistic but ultimately ineffective in losing weight. One of the keys to successful weight loss is to exercise smart, not long.

We conclude with Part 3, "Living Flipped" (because I already believe in your ability to be successful), with Chapter 11, "'Oh No, I Just Gained Five Pounds Back.'" In this section, I urge you to under-

LEARN FROM YOUR
FAILURES—AND YOUR
SUCCESSES

EXERCISE EFFECTIVELY
IN A LIMITED AMOUNT
OF TIME

stand that at some point while living flipped, you will probably regain some weight. First, I'll outline many situations or issues that may arise that could lead you to reverse the flip. Once you are aware of these potential pitfalls, your chances of lifelong success are ensured because you'll understand how to manage, outmaneuver, and ultimately avoid these traps and continue with your success. Second, I'll explore the emotional reality of what it feels like to regain some weight. Understanding your feelings when this happens to you could be a critical point in determining whether you stay flipped for life. Almost every person I have ever worked with has at some point gained a little weight back. Notice I said a "little" weight. It's usually in the range of five pounds. If you follow my lead, you, too, will be able to get back on track once the scale moves a little north.

So, clear your mind. Focus on the positive and your desire to live a longer, happier, healthier, thinner life. You *can* start from now and make a brand-new ending. Now is the time to lay that groundwork for a new future. I know you can do it—just *flip the switch*.

JIM KARAS

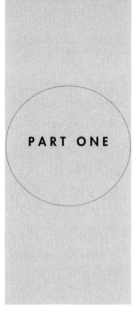

PART ONE

It Can Happen to You

1 Believe in the Flip

Countless times each year, I receive the same phone call. One of my clients will leave a message on my voice mail similar to the following: "I can't believe it. I got on the scale this morning and I am down over nine pounds. I haven't lost this much weight in years and I feel great. For the first time, I believe I can really lose weight, but I am nervous. Please call me and tell me that this is for real. Please tell me that I can keep this up and lose even more weight. Please tell me that I won't gain it all back. Please tell me that this is not a fluke. Please call me!"

Believing in yourself is the first step to flipping the switch. My goal in this chapter is for you to once and for all believe in the fact that you can succeed at weight loss. At the moment, you probably don't believe you can succeed. Undoubtedly, you have attempted weight loss dozens—or if you are like me, hundreds—of times in the past. I bet there isn't a diet that you haven't experienced. I tried fasting, food combining, high protein, low protein, high carbs, no carbs, and skipping meals to name but a few. Did you really believe that you would succeed in losing weight on *any* of these plans, or was trying these diets just an act of throwing up your hands and saying, "At this point, I'll try just about anything. I've got to do something."

That's where you made your first mistake. Yes, of course, these diets were nutty, but you were desperate, and desperate individuals embrace all types of wild strategies. Your error was not in trying; your error was that you did not believe in yourself. Instead, you believed in what turned out to be a quick fix that had no lasting results. Even if these programs had some basis in fact, you were doomed to fail. To succeed you must believe in your ability to be

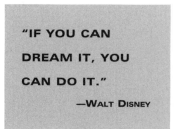

"IF YOU CAN DREAM IT, YOU CAN DO IT."
—WALT DISNEY

successful. You undertook each of these diet plans believing that you alone were not strong enough to triumph; instead, you put your faith into a plan that didn't work. Doubting yourself is a recipe for failure. In *Flip the Switch* I am going to teach you to believe in yourself and consequently break the cycle of starting and stopping, starting and stopping, which guarantees failure. I realize that you rationalized your behavior by saying, "At least I'm trying something." And, as I said, I don't fault you for trying, but I know (and I'm sure you do as well) that approaching the complicated task of weight loss requires more than a hot, trendy diet or a celebrity-endorsed exercise program. To begin the process, you must first believe in your ability to succeed. You can allow fear and doubt to enter your mind, but you *cannot* let them take control.

Do you recall your American history? What did FDR urge the American public to realize in his first inaugural address in March 1933 at the height of the Great Depression? By stressing "the only thing we have to fear is fear itself," FDR was able to convince Americans that they could achieve economic victory if they successfully avoided being paralyzed by fear and doubt. In other words, the president was stating the obvious. Don't allow fear and doubt to prevent you from taking action. That same attitude applies to any challenge you undertake and that includes weight loss. Don't be afraid to believe in the power of yourself. By doing so you will be creating a foundation upon which to build success in many areas of your life, not only weight loss.

Comfortable?

Look at it this way. Right now, you are probably comfortable *not* believing in your ability to flip. You are, however, unhappy with your weight. Holding this book in your hands indicates that you have a desire to change. Change is scary. We are all most comfortable with those issues, experiences, and situations that are familiar. Why do you think we keep going back to the same restaurants, the same vacation spots, the same stores? We know what to expect. No surprises, no discomfort. But once we entertain a desire to change, or directly experience change, our comfort level begins to diminish.

When I was a student at the University of Pennsylvania's Wharton School, I remember hating statistics. Just the thought of this class on Tuesdays and Thursdays made me sick. So what did I do? Well, I frequently skipped class, refused to open the book, and constantly had a sense of agitation about the class—classic avoidance. Halfway through the semester, at the last possible moment, I dropped the class. What a sense of relief I felt as I walked back to my fraternity house and realized that I no longer had to deal with the "statistics" issue. This lasted about two days. Then it dawned on me that it was a required class. I needed it to graduate. Sure, I was relieved that I didn't have to deal with it at that moment, but I was not very happy when I realized that I had created only a temporary solution. Next semester I had to take statistics again. Had I been smarter, and braver, I would have realized that I was already halfway through with this "torture." So why did I drop this class when half the pain was over? I didn't believe in my ability to succeed. I doubted myself and withdrew from the class.

The same principles apply to weight loss. How many times have you said to yourself, "I'm going to start losing weight this Monday"— or next month, or (the big one) January first? You take the pressure off at the moment, and that gives you a sense of relief, but the problem hasn't been solved. If you are overweight, the sooner you begin to deal with that issue, the faster the weight will come off and the better you will feel.

Draw from Your Inner Power

Start believing deep down inside that you can flip the switch and lose weight. Go deep within yourself all the way to your emotional epicenter. Draw from those feelings that are deep within you. You must begin to accept and believe in the power of the human mind to foster change. To reinforce this point, consider the following studies.

The Body and the Mind Work Together

The human mind is an extremely potent mechanism and researchers have long noted its power. In January 2002, the *American Journal of Psychiatry* reported on Andrew Leuchter and his colleagues at UCLA, who performed brain scans on fifty-one patients suffering from major depression. Half the patients were taking antidepressants and the other half had been given a placebo (a substance having no effect). Surprisingly, an equal number of people in *both* groups reported feeling better. More important, though, was the fact that the brain scans of those individuals who received the placebo recorded significant increased neurological activity in the brain's prefrontal cortex, the part of the brain that regulates mood, among other things. "What this study shows for the first time is that people who get better on placebo have a change in brain function, just as surely as people who get better on medication," stated Leuchter. Simply put, those individuals on the placebo believed that they should be feeling better and made their body physically respond to enable it to feel better. Both the body and the mind had a similar goal and worked in tandem to achieve that goal.

There have been numerous accounts of the power of the mind contributing to a changed physical state—such as individuals with multiple personalities being diabetic in one personality and free of diabetes in another. The power of the mind is awesome. Believe me, you can tap into that mental power just as others have done.

What follows is additional recent research that supports the power of "belief." Jane Ogden, Ph.D., a health psychologist at Guys Kings and St. Thomas' School of Medicine in London, studied groups of women, those who successfully lost weight and kept it off and those who didn't. She found two interesting points. First, the women who believed their weight problem was a function of their behavior, as in their eating and exercise habits, and not a result of external factors such as genes or metabolism, were "more successful at losing pounds because they believed that *they* were in control of their weight—and, therefore, believed they could lose weight." So, if you first take responsibility and believe that your behavior has led you to be overweight, then, if you believe that it is in your power to change that behavior, you can succeed.

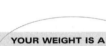

Second, she found that "once you believe weight loss success is possible, you'll feel less intimidated by challenges you encounter along the way." This is the mistake I made with my statistics class. I didn't believe that I would succeed, felt intimidated, and quit. Had I believed, I would have stayed, passed, and prevailed. You can do the same with weight loss.

Wipe Out the "Mental Graffiti"

Briefly look at this the opposite way. What does doubt do to your ability to succeed at weight loss? I refer to this doubt as "mental graffiti." This is clutter, a cacophony of doubt that is flowing through the brain: "I can't lose weight. I can't succeed. I can't stay on my program. I can't eat the right foods. I can't exercise. I can't look better and feel better. I can't even stop gaining weight." When negative phrases like these ricochet through your mind, the *c* word—*can't*—is winning. Here's where I start to get really tough with my clients. The first time I hear the *c* word I say, "No, no, no, we are not saying *can't*. Substitute the *can't* with *can*. That's a *c* word I can accept." Now repeat after me. Say *I can lose weight. I can succeed. I can stay on my program. I can eat the right foods.* It's time to wipe the negative mental graffiti off the board, start with a clean slate, and begin the flipping process.

Go Back in Time

Let's start at *your* beginning; that is, your childhood. I want you to think about your first impression of your body. Don't overly intellectualize this impression. When you go back to your childhood and recall your perception of your body, what is the first thought that comes into your head? This will be your first "exercise" toward flipping the switch, and you thought I would probably have you doing push-ups, didn't you? It is important to begin with a mental exercise because, as you have just seen, ultimately one's mind-set contributes far more to success at weight loss than one's physical behavior.

Fear of failure is a conditioned response. The probability is great that you were conditioned to feel a certain way about your body and that conditioning has stayed within you. What I'm going to assist you with is the letting go of that past negative conditioning. Okay, let's get started building a new positive mental imprint.

To help you to reach that point, I want you to get out a pen and complete the following sentence: *My very first impression of my body was . . .* (Use the space provided on page 14.)

RELEASE THE NEGATIVE
CONDITIONING

BELIEVE
IN THE
FLIP

13

BELIEVE IN THE FLIP

My very first impression of my
body was . . .

_____

_____

_____

_____

_____

_____

_____

_____

_____

_____

_____

_____

_____

Here's what I wrote about myself: *My very first impression of my body was that it was plump. People referred to me as "husky," "potbellied," "nonathletic." I couldn't run very fast, I didn't play sports, the thought of gym class made me sick, and I never, I repeat never, wanted to take my shirt off at the beach.*

To this day, this first impression lives within me. I know now that it is not true, but I do remember what that feeling was like and, honestly, it hurt. It hurt a lot.

Pause for a moment. Look at what you have written. Reflect on your comments for a few minutes. Let your mind drift back in time. Recall those feelings. This exercise probably will be painful, but please don't feel that I am attempting one of those "no pain, no gain" strategies. That's not my intent. It's important that you start at the beginning. By recalling these first impressions, though painful, we begin the emotional rebuilding process.

During childhood you formed the first impression of your physical self. First impressions tend to remain in our mind's eye. My first impression of my physical self was a negative one. So, it is that impression that I needed to overcome to ultimately succeed at weight loss. In time, we will also look at examples of individuals who began their lives with positive impressions of their body, but then that feeling changed as they proceeded through life and gained weight.

Now I want you to complete the following sentence in the space provided on page 15: *My current impression of my body is . . .*

Once again, using myself as an example, this is what I would write today: *My current impression of my body is that I am strong, lean, able to lift my kids high in the air (and don't forget, they keep growing). I can run down the block or up a flight of stairs without being out of breath. I open my closet and choose what to wear not by what will fit but by what will make me feel good, and, yes, now I can take my shirt off at the beach!*

Do you see how different my first impression is from the current one? Please bear in mind that it took a long time mentally to develop and accept this new one. I had to work very hard to break with my initial impressions of my body. Compare your two descriptions. How different is your first impression from the present one? In working with clients I have learned that people generally fall into one of two categories when answering these questions.

Some fall into category 1, "Lifelong Strugglers." These individuals remember *always* being overweight. Whether they truly were overweight or were connected to a parent or another individual who led them to believe this was the case, the fact remains that these individuals have had a lifelong struggle with this issue. I am one of these people. I remember being overweight, and even though I have developed the tools (both mentally and physically) to keep the weight off, I will always vividly recall that feeling, though that no longer is my reality.

The other category includes individuals who wake up one day, probably in their late thirties, forties, or fifties, and find themselves carrying around an additional twenty-five pounds or more on their bodies. These are what I call the "Slow Gainers." Whenever I or one of my staff conducts a new client interview, we ask the prospective client to fill out an information form that requests his or her body weight over the years. Generally, we see a pattern of slow, consistent weight gain each year. These people say to us, "I just don't know how this happened. I never had a weight problem. I was one hundred and twenty pounds for many years. Now I struggle to stay under one hundred and fifty-five. What's happened to me?"

BELIEVE IN THE FLIP

My current impression of my body is . . .

Please read both of these category descriptions carefully, no matter which one you fall into, for the following reason: You will be asked to complete a number of written exercises to create your own personal "profile" as I do with clients at our initial consultation. If you skip over these descriptions, you may wind up skipping over important questions. The exercises/questions in the Slow Gainer section, for instance, should also be addressed by individuals who fall into the Lifelong Struggler category.

Frequently this individual will require a different coaching strategy from a weight-loss consultant than the Lifelong Struggler. Why? Slow Gainers possess little or no familiarity with weight loss. Teaching tools and a protocol, such as eating less and exercising effectively, to someone who has never dealt with these instructions can be more difficult than training Lifelong Strugglers, who have been around these tools and protocols for years.

Into which category do you fall—Lifelong Struggler or Slow Gainer? I want you to note these two categories because, as I just explained, it is necessary to take a slightly different psychological approach to ultimately lead both categories to flip. Of course, it is possible that some individuals do not clearly fall into one of these two categories, but from my experience most do. Understanding these two categories will also enable you to be more empathetic in dealing with a loved one, friend, or family member who struggles with weight loss, so don't skip one category and jump to the next even if you firmly believe you have already determined *your* category. Read the descriptions below carefully and understand the dynamics of each. It will increase your knowledge of and compassion for all of those who struggle with weight loss.

Category 1: Lifelong Strugglers

Lifelong Strugglers such as myself *always* remember being overweight. I cannot remember a time from my very early childhood until my twenties that I was not about to start yet another attempt at weight loss. I actually remember running in place in my family room (I was too intimidated to do it in public) or trying to jump rope in a desperate attempt to shed some pounds.

I even bought a product called the Wonder Weighted Belt, which claimed to reduce your abdominal area by three inches in no time. As directed, I attached myself to a doorknob, and with the Wonder Weighted Belt strapped around my waist performed some ridiculous exercises. I was devastated when it didn't work. Lifelong Strugglers have had a negative perception of their bodies right from the beginning. Hundreds of people who have discussed this specific issue with me have said they felt they were always overweight. They stressed that they vividly recall negative comments regarding their appearance and those comments stayed with them. Please realize that I am not trying to single out parents, but frequently those remarks came from either a mother or a father. In most instances, these parents didn't intentionally mean to inflict mental anguish on their children, but many times their negative remarks stemmed from their own internal unhappiness and they projected this dissatisfaction on their children. (I will go into much more detail on this subject in Chapter 9, "'I'm a Woman.'"). The child becomes an adult, hangs on to the conditioning, doubts herself, stays overweight, and becomes a Lifelong Struggler. What can a Lifelong Struggler, now an adult, do to overcome this conditioning?

Memories

You begin by recalling your childhood in detail. Yes, this is painful, but necessary. Were you really overweight, perhaps obese, as a child, or were you simply carrying around a few extra pounds? There are many adults today who were perfectly healthy children but were led to *believe* they had to diet and were overweight. Today, these adults are angry. They are angry because the message that they received was false and that false message inflicted tremendous psychological damage. Quite often, the parents or people who led them to believe that they were overweight were raised by individuals who inflicted similar behavior on them. The psychiatric community calls this "classic repetition." Rather than learn from the mistakes and pain of their own childhood, they, too, repeated the same with their children—in this case, perhaps you. It doesn't necessarily mean that they didn't love you; they were simply following the negative conditioning they had been exposed to in their own childhood.

It's quite possible that a Lifelong Struggler started out perfectly healthy and at an appropriate weight, but after a few years, the effects of these negative comments prevailed. An overweight child with eating and exercise issues was created.

Of course, it is entirely possible that you actually were overweight. However, keep in mind that years ago there statistically weren't many kids who were classified as being overweight.

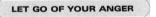

WERE THERE MANY OVERWEIGHT KIDS IN YOUR GRADE-SCHOOL CLASSES?

I don't remember a lot of other kids who had a weight problem like mine. I distinctly remember being part of a minority. *Parenting* magazine reported that "in 1960, only 4 percent of children ages 6 to 11 were seriously overweight, according to federal statistics. By 1980 it was 7 percent. It jumped again by the early '90s, and by 1999 the figure was 13 percent." Additionally, the *Journal of the American Medical Association* noted that "between 1986 and 1998, the number of overweight children increased by more than 50 percent among white children, but by more than 120 percent among African Americans and Hispanics." This statistic does not include teenagers who have been gaining weight at an astonishing rate. Whenever I take my daughter or son to the playground or attend a school function, I am always amazed at the number of overweight children. If this trend continues unchecked, the United States will face a major health crisis by the end of the first quarter of the twenty-first century as these children become adults.

Weight and Depression

For now, let's assume that you actually were overweight as a child for whatever reason. Frequently, overweight children grow into angry adults who turn that anger inward. There is another word for anger turned inward—*depression.* Consequently, there's a high probability that you are angry and depressed about being overweight. You are also perhaps angry at the individual or individuals who made you feel bad about being overweight. It's even possible that you keep the weight on and refuse to flip as a way of getting back at that individual. Losing weight would constitute a "change." Yes, either consciously or subconsciously, you continue to hold on to the weight as a way of striking back at that individual, or you use it to avoid dealing with other issues in your life, such as personal relationships or career goals.

LET GO OF YOUR ANGER

Psychiatrists have long noted these behavior patterns among overweight patients. Right now, if you are holding on to your anger, the only person you are hurting is *you*. The individuals responsible for this anger may be gone, or elderly, or most likely don't even remember what they said to you, yet you are allowing their mental picture of you to prevail. This emotional anger is preventing you from believing that you *can* succeed at weight loss. It is *their* image of you that is still defining you today. You need to cast this aside as you approach losing weight. After all, whose mental picture should prevail—theirs or yours?

So, I want you, as a Lifelong Struggler, to complete the following sentence: *You, (insert the name), made me feel bad about my appearance . . .* (Use the space provided at right.)

Once again, this is what I wrote: *You, Mr. Junior High School Gym Teacher, made me feel bad about my appearance and my ability to play sports. You teased me in front of my friends, made me hate sports even more, and for a long period of time turned me off to any physical activity. Being thirteen years old was bad enough without you making it worse.*

Even as I write this it brings back those old feelings, but I adamantly refuse to let this old mental graffiti prevail. This is not easy for me, nor will it be for you. You have to dredge up feelings that you have long buried. Try. These feelings of anger will not be pleasant, but they can be the root of your inability to believe you can flip. Take the anger that you have bottled up within you and use it as a catalyst to create change. Simply put, take the negative, the anger, and turn it into a positive force for constructive change.

Parents: Be Careful with What You Say

For those of you who are parents or are frequently around children, a cautionary note: Realize that you

BELIEVE IN THE FLIP

You, (insert the name), made me feel bad about my appearance . . .

are contributing to the formulation of your child's beliefs *every day.* Be aware, very aware, that what you say, how you phrase it, and how you respond to situations and individuals are being cataloged by the child. My wife and I are very careful in our household about using certain words or phrases. We don't use the words *fat* or *overweight,* especially around our five-and-a-half-year-old daughter, as she hears everything within a six-mile range. Whenever my kids—or for that matter, any children—are within earshot, I ask people not to talk about weight loss. This can be tough because, naturally, weight loss is the principal topic about which most people want to pick my brain. When we talk about what Daddy does for a living, we tell our kids that I help people eat healthy food and exercise.

Can you just see the impact of telling your children that Daddy helps people lose weight? Immediately, regardless of their size, they would look at themselves and ask, "Do I need to lose weight? Am I overweight?" Certainly this is one of the last things parents should desire for their children. Don't create an image in children that causes them to fixate on an issue that may or may not be an issue. Avoid creating an obsession. Remember, children do so want to please their parents. They are constant observers of adult behavior and frequently mirror that behavior.

Decades ago, the psychiatric community didn't urge us to be careful with what we said and did in front of children. Today, we realize the powerful impression we make on the young. Eating issues tend to begin very, very early in life. Body images are formed early. Please exercise caution with regard to comments about body weight when you are around *all* children. Trust me, I didn't like being told I had a "cute" potbelly. I realized this was negative commentary. Adults laughed at me and hurt my feelings; I ended up eating even more.

This prompts me to bring up one more point regarding parents and children. Overweight parents should realize that they may be raising overweight children. I am not going to go into the genes/metabolism discussion at this time because I've devoted Chapter 6, "'I Don't Have the Right Genes or Metabolism,'" to this issue. Just be cognizant that what you are doing now is being mirrored by your children. Children want to please their parents. If that means sitting around the house watching television and eating chips, they'll do it. If it means running around the block and eating apples, they'll do it. So much of their programming, especially in the early years, rests with you. Kids are terrific at copying. It's how they learn. Recall the expression "Monkey see, monkey do."

We become "imprinted" with certain behavior patterns at a very early age. According to Judith Sills, Ph.D., the author of *Excess Baggage,* these imprints then become a powerful bridge between mind and body. "It's taken years for your mind to build its scaffolding of tricks and worries," she states, so "it takes time to dismantle." Realize this. Don't pile that "excess baggage" on your child.

≪

Okay, Lifelong Struggler, review your three exercises. You should have written at least one sentence each on your past and present impressions of your appearance and the individual(s) who led you to believe these impressions were true. Look back and reread what you wrote. These exercises will become the foundation of believing you can once and for all flip the switch.

You also have to start talking about these factors. Though painful, it is necessary that you allow these issues to bubble to the surface. For years you have used your body weight and/or food to mask these feelings and issues and have kept them bottled up inside yourself. Now I want you to intentionally open the "wound." Yes, I call this a wound, one that never really healed. Instead, it amassed scar tissue around it. The scar tissue keeps the wound from being readily apparent, somewhat numbing the pain but also preventing complete healing. Chip away at that scar tissue and start the healing process once and for all.

START TALKING TO OTHER FAMILY MEMBERS

You might consider discussing these factors with a sibling or another relative who was around your home when you were growing up. Perhaps he or she observed certain behavior patterns and some of the dynamics of your family relationships. If so, you will be armed with additional data to better understand your present-day feelings and attitudes.

You might also consider some professional therapy, which can be tremendously beneficial for certain individuals. I can attest that therapy helped me dramatically in every area of my life, from my marriage to how I interact with my children, to my friendships, and to my work/career. I was not the only one who benefited. All those around me did as well. Why wouldn't anyone want to better understand their feelings, attitudes, and behavior? That's what therapy is all about. You gain important insights as to why you react the way you do to people, places, and things.

If you feel that you'd benefit from professional therapy, don't automatically reject it because it is too expensive. It doesn't need to be. Many counseling centers all over the country are set up on a sliding scale, where you pay what you can afford. Or you might consider organizations such as Overeaters Anonymous. Being around other individuals who share your struggle allows you to share your issues and journeys. You learn from their struggle, they learn from yours, and mentally that's a big plus. You'll also learn that you are not alone.

Category 2: Slow Gainers

Slow Gainers began their lives, and most likely the early part of their adulthood, with positive impressions of their bodies. They were probably very close to their ideal body weight for their height and age. These people frequently use expressions such as "I never had to watch what I ate," "I never had a weight problem," "I used to really like my body and how I looked." Slowly, and somewhat subtly, a change began.

Ask a College Student

This weight gain might have occurred as early as college. A Tufts University research study says that "thirty-two percent of all college students reported a 'decline' in their body image during their freshman year: forty percent of college women at an appropriate weight perceive that they are overweight." Think about that: Close to half of the women at an appropriate weight think of themselves as being overweight. Attitudes such as these could trigger the Slow-Gainer pattern to form as they start a vicious dieting cycle while the weight creeps up. So that I am clear, these women didn't initially have a weight problem but created one as they began to diet, then regain the weight, diet, then regain even more weight until ultimately they had a significant weight problem.

HAVE YOU SEEN A
PATTERN OF SLOW,
CONSISTENT WEIGHT
GAIN EACH YEAR?

Postpartum Pounds

For women, a weight gain frequently happens after having children. They gained weight, as they should have with the pregnancy, but after the birth, they are unable to shed those last few pounds. Then, with each subsequent pregnancy, the process repeats itself until the cumulative effect is that they are permanently twenty, thirty, or more pounds over their prepregnancy weight.

The Slow Creep Up

Another scenario that many of us are familiar with goes like this: As men and women proceed through their twenties and thirties they become more sedentary and begin to lose lean muscle tissue (which slows their basal metabolism, or daily caloric burning), but continue to consume the same number of calories they consumed when they were younger. Long hours at the office, the juggling of a family and children, business or social dinners, or the aforementioned lack of physical activity led them to slowly, each year, put on additional pounds. By gaining slowly but steadily year after year, many Americans will find themselves thirty, forty, fifty, sixty, seventy, or more pounds overweight within a relatively brief period of time. This unfortunate trend will be examined in greater detail in subsequent chapters.

Many people, furthermore, don't understand why they have gained this weight. I can't tell you the number of times I've asked clients, "How did this weight gain happen?" only to have them reply, "I don't know." The process was often so subtle, and since the same thing was happening to their friends or spouses, they didn't notice it until one day they couldn't keep up with their kids at the playground or didn't fit into their favorite outfit or were shocked by their reflection in the mirror.

Now reread your answer to the first exercise, *"My very first impression of my body was . . ."* Then look at your answer to the second exercise, *"My current impression of my body is . . ."* Compare the two. Your assignment is to determine what happened in between the two impressions. To do so, I want you to complete the sentence for each appropriate decade in the spaces provided on the following pages.

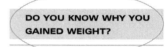

DO YOU KNOW WHY YOU GAINED WEIGHT?

BELIEVE IN THE FLIP

In my twenties, my highest weight was _____ and my lowest weight was _____. This is what I was doing with regard to eating and exercise . . .

_____

_____

_____

_____

In my thirties, my highest weight was _____ and my lowest weight was _____. This is what I was doing with regard to eating and exercise . . .

_____

_____

_____

_____

In my forties, my highest weight was _____ and my lowest weight was _____. This is what I was doing with regard to eating and exercise . . .

_____

_____

At my present age, my response would be: *Presently, my highest weight is 174 and my lowest weight is 169. I am performing strength and resistance exercise three to four times a week for approximately 45 minutes. This includes a 10-minute cardiovascular warmup. I am eating a diet high in lean protein, vegetables, and fruits and try to stay in the 2,000–2,200-calorie-a-day range to maintain my weight and go down to between 1,500–1,600 calories a day when I need to lose some weight.*

Just as my weight-loss management firm creates a profile of a new client's weight at the initial interview, you, too, have just created a profile of your weight over the years and the relevant behaviors associated with that weight. Most important, this exercise gives you information to help illustrate why you are currently struggling with your weight. Look long and hard—and objectively—at your responses and draw the appropriate conclusions.

Why Answering Some Questions Will Help You Flip

Exercise 4 should also be completed by the Lifelong Struggler. I know that just like me you've tried numerous weight-loss programs over the years. Examine what worked for you, even for a brief period of time, and what didn't. This is basically a form of research. You need to find out what was happening and what your eating/exercise behavior consisted of at those times in order to fully understand why you have struggled with your weight over the years.

Similarly, exercise 3, where I asked you to identify the person or persons who made you feel bad about your body weight, is an appropriate exercise not only for Lifelong Strugglers but for some Slow Gainers as well. Often someone is presently making you feel awful about the way you look. It could be a spouse, parent, sibling, or coworker. You need to learn to deal with the anger/guilt that undoubtedly is associated with those feelings. I have gone out socially with some couples for whom the tension surrounding the body-weight issue was enormous. I have watched people purposely load their bread with butter and order huge quantities of food just to irritate their spouses. I know of one woman who has lost more than twenty pounds whose overweight husband brings home her favorite goodies from the bakery. Please fill in that sentence if there is someone who is making you feel bad. Then try to determine why the person is doing this and discuss your feelings with him or her. It can make a significant difference in your ability to lose weight and will contribute to a positive mind-set.

As I said earlier, ultimately you are the one in control of what you eat and whether or not you exercise. The purpose of exercise 3 is to determine if someone else continues to thwart your ability to succeed at weight loss. If no such person exists, then this isn't an issue.

An Epidemic in Front of Our Eyes

Regardless of whether you are a Lifelong Struggler or a Slow Gainer, you are faced with a similar situation as you begin this weight-loss journey. According to the most recent statistics, more than 64.5 percent of the American population is presently overweight and almost 20 percent are categorized as obese (more than 20 percent over their optimal body weight). An article in the *Journal of the American Medical Association* stated that the number of obese Americans has increased by 49 percent since 1991. According to William Dietz, director of the Division of Nutrition and Physical Activity at the Centers for Disease Control and Prevention in Atlanta, "A rise of such a

In my fifties, my highest weight was _____ and my lowest weight was _____. This is what I was doing with regard to eating and exercise . . .

Do this for each decade until you arrive at your present age. Then, conclude with the following:

Presently, my highest weight is _____ and my lowest weight is _____. Currently, this is what I am doing with regard to eating and exercise . . .

magnitude [in obesity] is a unique observation in the annals of chronic disease. We're seeing an epidemic of a chronic disease right in front of our eyes."

More than 64.5 percent represents a *majority* of our population. That's correct, a majority of the American population is now overweight. If you are overweight, you are not alone. Those at an appropriate body weight are in the *minority;* therefore, millions of Americans, whether Lifelong Strugglers or Slow Gainers, need to lose weight. Why haven't they? We all know that there is no shortage of diet and exercise programs available in the marketplace. One can barely turn on the television, listen to the radio, or open a newspaper or magazine without being bombarded with one extravagant weight-loss promise after another. Polls indicate that at any one time a significant number of Americans state that they either are on a diet or should be on a diet. Year after year, losing weight is the number one New Year's resolution. Yet we remain an overweight nation. Why don't diets perform as well as they claim to, and why are so many Americans on them or believe that they should be?

Don't Go for a Gimmick

The vast majority of diet plans don't succeed because they are based on some sort of gimmick. Yes, it is true that these gimmicks, which frequently advocate totally eliminating a food or food group, can *briefly* change an individual's body weight, because most of these diet plans quickly deplete the body's water balance, which does cause the scale to go down. Your goal is to shed fat, not water. Once you eliminate the gimmick, the weight returns as the water returns. It was water that was shed, not fat. Remember all the times you recall losing five pounds in a brief period of time and gaining it back just as quickly? What you lost was water, not fat. Such weight-loss gimmicks never succeed in permanently keeping weight off.

Second, most diet plans are predicated on incorrect information. Here is an example. A bestselling weight-loss book claims carrots will make you fat. Now, mind you, there is not a single shred of scientific evidence that supports this theory. In reality, the fact is that carrots have very few calories, are packed with vitamins, and in no way contribute to the so-called spiking of one's insulin level. I repeat, there is

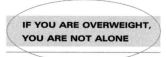
IF YOU ARE OVERWEIGHT, YOU ARE NOT ALONE

not one serious bit of scientific research that points to carrots as the reason why Americans are overweight. Yet I constantly see people pick carrots out of their salads. Are carrots the culprit? No, but the individuals picking those carrots out of their salads should reconsider the salad dressing, which usually contains hundreds of calories, that they've put on top of a few harmless carrots. Eat all the carrots you want without dressing. Trust me, you won't gain a pound.

Keep in mind, this is just one of the nutty weight-loss theories out there. There are so many others. Don't forget the "Hollywood Miracle Diet" that claims you will lose ten pounds in two days, the "Cabbage Soup Diet," the "Grapefruit Diet," and the "Eat All You Want and Lose Weight" diet—right! "Eat All You Want and Lose Weight" is a great marketing phrase. Can it happen? You tell me.

Furthermore, few if any of the current weight-loss programs realistically address weight loss as a lifelong plan. To be comprehensive and successful, weight-loss plans must incorporate proper eating, effective exercise, and, most important, the belief in your ability to succeed. To change your relationship with your body, you have to think about it before you can do it. As you are thinking about it, start believing that you can succeed.

Being Overweight Is Not a Fact of Life

You cannot accept being overweight as a fact of life. Also, it's not the result of aging. Though, as you will learn in subsequent chapters, aging can contribute to weight gain, that process can be easily reversed. Turn to Chapter 8, "'I Hate to Exercise,'" if you need that information immediately. But for now, as you are learning to believe in yourself, realize that you can lose weight at any point in life. *Believe me!* For that matter, at any point in life you can succeed at almost any task or goal, with the possible exceptions of being a teen model or an Olympic athlete. Why do you think "It's never too late" became an adage?

Whether you are a Lifelong Struggler or a Slow Gainer, you must firmly believe that you can succeed at weight loss. Say that to yourself right now. Say it out loud. Write it down. Type it on your computer screen. *I can succeed at weight loss.* Remember the client who

NO, YOU CAN'T REALLY LOSE TEN POUNDS IN JUST TWO DAYS

SUCCESSFUL WEIGHT-LOSS PLANS ARE COMPREHENSIVE

BELIEVE IN THE FLIP

I believed in my ability to be successful in achieving my goal of . . .

_____

_____

_____

_____

_____

_____

_____

_____

_____

_____

_____

_____

_____

_____

was losing weight but needed constant reassurance that the loss would continue? I want you to consider yourself "in process," too. Being "in process" means that you are always examining the many psychological and physiological reasons that have prevented you from flipping. Please don't think that you only have to flip once. It's truly an ongoing process. Remember, I still consider myself in process. Yes, there are times I want to turn to food and I get tired of exercise. But I hold to my belief that I can live my life as a healthier, thinner person, and I use that belief to get me through a difficult time. You, too, must subscribe to that belief. Without that attitude, I cannot guide you to success. Again, the key is believing in yourself.

Here is the next exercise to help you to believe in yourself. I want you to think for just a moment about some other aspect of your life when you believed in yourself and your ability to attain a goal and succeeded in achieving that goal; then complete this sentence in the space provided at left: _I believed in my ability to be successful in achieving my goal of . . ._

Now, describe that time when you believed in yourself—in your ability to be a good partner, spouse, parent, or employee. You may have believed in your ability to decorate a room, throw a surprise birthday party, or coach a Little League team. Whatever your goal might have been, I am certain that you believed in your ability to achieve that goal and ultimately were successful in the endeavor: When you _believed in yourself,_ you achieved your goal.

Once again, using myself as an example, I would complete this thought by saying: _I believed in my ability to be successful in achieving my goal of owning my own business. I was never very comfortable working for other people and knew that I wanted to have total control over my career path._

The Fear Flipper

A few years ago, I interviewed a new client. In his middle fifties, he was extremely overweight, had both high blood pressure and high cholesterol levels, and was essentially a heart attack waiting to happen. During our conversation, it was quickly apparent to me that this individual truly did not possess the desire to be successful at weight loss. As we chatted, he repeatedly remarked that he was doing this because his wife, kids, and physician nagged him to lose weight. When I asked, "Have you ever tried to lose weight in the past?," he replied, "Sure, but I always found exercise boring and I can't stand eating that 'rabbit food.' When I get home from work, I need 'good food' to fill me up." I knew I had a challenge on my hands.

He agreed to work out three times a week and to record and submit daily food journals. During the next three months, he managed to shed ten pounds; however, he still needed to lose at least an additional forty pounds to reach a healthy weight. My staff informed me that he frequently skipped workout sessions and stopped maintaining his food journal after only a few weeks.

Unfortunately, the predicted heart attack occurred, and my client needed a quadruple bypass. After he recovered from the surgery and had obtained medical clearance, he resumed his program with my firm—with a vengeance. He no longer canceled his training sessions. He dutifully monitored his caloric intake in a food diary and faxed it to my office. He subsequently lost an additional twenty pounds. Obviously, the heart attack and surgery had not only frightened him but motivated him. Unfortunately, his new exemplary behavior was short-lived—it lasted approximately three months. Then old habits prevailed. He once again started missing exercise sessions, resumed his unhealthy eating patterns, and, you guessed it, subsequently regained all the weight he had lost. What happened?

My impression is that once he was no longer afraid he might die, his belief in his ability to succeed at his weight-loss program disappeared. He had flipped temporarily out of fear, an external stimuli, but once that fear had ceased, he flipped back. We desperately tried to get him back on track. He said he wasn't interested. Obviously, he

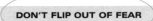
DON'T FLIP OUT OF FEAR

had never truly believed in his ability to succeed. He had been frightened and that fear fueled his flip. He is what I call a "Fear Flipper."

A considerable body of research supports this type of behavior. Jaylan Turkkan, Ph.D., chief of behavioral sciences research at the National Institute on Drug Abuse, says, "Fear almost never works in the long term. In the short term, people get rattled and try to change, but eventually the fear goes away and the desire for immediate pleasure takes over." Clearly, this is the case with millions of Americans.

The Special-Event Flipper

My weight-loss management firm, Jim Karas Personal Training, LLC, has had dozens of clients who, prior to a special event—say, a milestone birthday (fifty is a big one), anniversary, reunion, or bar mitzvah—will embark on a major weight-loss program. They become model clients, coupling intelligent eating with effective, consistent exercise. At the event, they look and feel great. If they were to complete exercise 2, "My current impression of my body is . . . ," just before the event, they would say that they feel and look the best they have in many, many years. They feel strong, confident, sexy, and once again in control of their weight and appearance. But time passes. The event no longer looms on the horizon. What happens? Invariably, the so-called bad behavior reappears, and the excess weight returns. Thus, once the event is over and the external motivation ceases, the ongoing belief that they can live flipped evaporates. The doubt resurfaces and the weight rapidly returns. A short time *after* the event, these individuals would write a far different ending to the sentence "My current impression of my body is . . ."

The "I'm Doing This for You, Not for Me" Flipper

Some people attempt weight loss for someone else, frequently a romantic interest. I have had numerous individuals, especially women, tell me that their spouse wants them to become more attractive by losing weight. I've heard of men who *claim* that they will date a woman if she is successful at losing weight. Teenagers have said to me that their mothers or fathers really want them to lose weight before going to college to be more attractive. One young man actually told me that

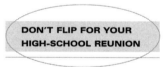
DON'T FLIP FOR YOUR
HIGH-SCHOOL REUNION

his father insisted he lose weight before going to college because he would be attending his father's alma mater. His father continued to be very involved with the school and didn't want his overweight son to embarrass him. He even went so far as to say that if his son didn't lose weight, he would not allow him to join his old fraternity. This young man was desperate and so very hurt by these comments.

If you are not losing weight for you, odds are you won't be successful. Why? Because you, not someone else, have to want it. You have to cut back on your calories. You have to exercise. The responsibility rests with you.

LOSE WEIGHT FOR YOURSELF

External versus Internal

Fear, a special event, and losing weight for someone else are external forces that motivate individuals to flip. In the preceding illustrations, these individuals did not arrive at the decision to lose weight on their own; rather, they let external situations dictate their behavior. Unfortunately, once the external situation changes, so does the behavior. I refer to this as the *external* versus *internal* motivation to flip. An external motivation rarely works in the long term. As I said, I have watched many men and women revert to their "bad" behavior after a heart attack and surgery, or some other life-threatening illness because they really had not internally arrived at the decision to change. They still doubted themselves; they didn't believe they could flip. I want you to decide this time to lose the weight for you—only for you. You must allow the motivation to come from within.

ONLY YOU CAN MAKE THE DECISION TO FLIP

Bernie and Manny

What follows is one of my favorite examples of internal motivation and its contribution to flipping the switch. Bernie played racquetball with his cousin Manny. After showering, as both men were dressing, Manny looked at Bernie and said, "When did you become such a fat f——?" Bernie laughed. They both laughed. Then, Bernie told me, he got in his car, looked down at his stomach, and agreed. "Yes, I have become a fat f——." After he got angry and cried a little, he drove home and called my firm. He decided then and there to flip. He has been an amazing success. To date, he has lost more than sixty pounds

BELIEVE IN THE FLIP—

When I am successful at losing even a little weight, I feel . . .

_____

_____

_____

_____

_____

_____

_____

_____

_____

_____

_____

_____

_____

_____

_____

and is a model client. You should see the smile on his face. He just projects great self-esteem and confidence since he took control of his weight. I believe he will stay flipped for life. Do you know why? It is because *he* made the decision to lose weight. Sure, Manny's comment was the catalyst, but Bernie decided to change the way he looked and felt and he followed through. *He* believed it. It worked. That desire to succeed came from within and turned into a reality.

Stay in Touch with Your Emotions

One tool that I have successfully employed with clients over the years to stimulate internal motivation is to ask them every month, "How are you feeling about your body?" I urge you to pose the same question to yourself. Constant monitoring of your current attitude toward your body is essential. As you begin the process of internally flipping, you need to stay in touch with the emotional changes that are also occurring. On the first of every month, once again complete the sentence, which I have provided for you in the back of the book: My current impression of my body is . . .

Whether you are a Lifelong Struggler or a Slow Gainer, you need to complete this sentence on a monthly basis. That way, your emotional and physical journeys will stay connected. If you notice that your entries begin to acquire a negative tone, or if you omit entries, you should be alert to make the necessary correction(s) to keep yourself from flipping off and allowing old feelings and impressions to resurface. (In the next chapter, I'll give you a tool for tracking these monthly entries.)

This leads us to the last two exercises of this chapter. I want you to complete the following sentence in the space provided on page 32 and be totally honest regarding your feelings: *When I am successful at losing even a little weight, I feel . . .*

My response is: *When I am successful at losing even a little weight, I feel in control. I feel that I am in control of my body and what goes into it. I feel that if I can lose just a little weight, I can accomplish anything.*

What did you write? Did your response approximate mine? I bet to a great extent it did. I honestly feel this way. For all of you reading this book, I believe that losing weight will give you the confidence and self-esteem to undertake additional goals and succeed. Give it a shot. After all, you have nothing to lose—nothing but weight!

This brings us to the final exercise of this chapter. I want you to complete the following sentence in the space provided at right: *When I gain weight, I feel . . .*

Here is my response: *When I gain weight, I feel horrible. I am so disappointed with myself. Why did I eat that? Why didn't I stop? Why am I letting cheese and salt change the way I look and feel? How am I going to get back to where I was? I feel a slight sense of panic and definitely get depressed.*

As I write this book, I am currently working with Dawnnie, a thirty-five-year-old woman, who has been appearing with me on ABC's *Good Morning America.* Dawnnie is a Lifelong Struggler who has decided she really wants to lose weight once and for all. When she began my program, she was five feet four inches tall and weighed 165 pounds. Dawnnie and I agree that she has about forty pounds to lose. It has been an interesting assignment. Dawnnie is working toward a master's degree in theater education. She is very pretty and has a great energy about her. When we talked about her weight loss, she made an interesting point. She said, "Even when I lose just a few

BELIEVE IN THE FLIP—

When I gain weight, I feel . . .

pounds, I feel so good about myself. I go out more. I'm happier. I have more energy. I just feel better." Similarly, she said, "When I gain weight, I totally retreat back into myself. I don't want to go out. I'm disappointed with myself. I feel a little lost." I find this occurs with most individuals. So, ask yourself, "How do I feel when I gain and lose weight?" I bet you already know the answer, but put it on paper and read it and reread it. By the way, in four months Dawnnie is already down twenty-five pounds. She is over halfway there!

Now that you've begun the process of believing you can flip the switch, we will begin moving to the next step. This step will present and demonstrate to you the power of visualization as a tool to reinforce and assist your belief in the flip.

≪

As you conclude "Believe in the Flip," I want you to come to the conclusion that you will succeed at weight loss. That is infinitely more valuable than if I simply advised you to "eat less, exercise more," which you know and I know is the numerical basis of weight loss. If eating less and exercising more were that easy, we would all have lost weight years ago. It requires so much more than a slogan such as "Just Say No to Food." It's just not that simple. What is keeping you and others from success at weight loss is your inability to reach the point where *you, you, you* believe that you can succeed at eating less and exercising more. Once you've come to terms with that emotional hurdle and discipline, the physical exercises will seem easy by comparison. Create your own private mantra, your theme song if you like, and just keep saying it over and over: "If they can do it, so can I. If they can do it, so can I."

IF THEY CAN DO IT, SO CAN I

PUTTING IT ALL TOGETHER TO FLIP

- To successfully lose weight and keep the weight off, it is necessary to first believe in your ability to be successful.
- You determined whether you are a Lifelong Struggler, a Slow Gainer, or perhaps some combination of the two.
- You participated in a number of mental exercises and recorded your responses. These exercises were designed to create awareness. There are no right or wrong answers. These answers represented *your* past and present relationship to body, food, and exercise.
- These exercises helped identify what has kept *you* from flipping.
- Don't be afraid of what the power of believing in yourself can generate. It will produce significant change and become the foundation upon which to build success for yourself in many areas of your life, not just weight loss.

2 Visualize the Flip

I had a client a number of years ago who really struggled with her weight. She conformed to the Slow-Gainer pattern of weight gain. She was close to seventy pounds overweight by the time she reached her middle fifties. Earlier in her life, weight had not been a problem. Now, nothing seemed to work. She said, "I've tried everything and never lost a pound!" She frequently repeated that lament. Then, one day as we were working together, her very trim daughter walked into the exercise room wearing a great-looking if tight-fitting cashmere coat. "It's too small," she said to her mother. "I wish this fit, but it is just too small. Don't you agree?" My client did, so her daughter left the room.

"I thought that coat was beautiful," I remarked. "Can't she just return it for a larger size?" My client said, "No, if you can believe it, that was a favorite coat of mine that I wore in my twenties." I instantly raced down the hall after the daughter, asked for the coat, and brought it back into the exercise room. I found a hanger, put it on the outside of the closet, and said, "This is going to be your motivation. I want you to look at this every time you are in this room and realize that you once fit into this coat. Let's make it your mission to fit into it once again."

One year later she could.

> "NOT EVERYTHING THAT IS FACED CAN BE CHANGED, BUT NOTHING CAN BE CHANGED UNTIL IT IS FACED."
>
> —JAMES BALDWIN

You are now "in process." That means you are starting to believe in your ability to once and for all flip the switch. To make this process easier and to keep continuing to believe in yourself, let me introduce you to an extremely powerful tool that will assist you and provide you with ongoing encouragement, motivation, and a daily dose of reinforcement. That tool is *visualization.* When we create a picture or goal in our mind, we are visualizing. According to Stephen Covey, author of *The Seven Habits of Highly Effective People,* "almost all world-class athletes and other peak performers visualize. They visualize their success whether it be tennis, golf, baseball—they see themselves actually winning the match, tournament or world series." This technique will give *you* the inspirational reinforcement necessary to carry through with your decision to lose weight. Start picturing yourself as a successful "loser" in your mind. Visualizing yourself as a success will strongly reinforce the belief that you can succeed.

CREATE A GOAL IN YOUR MIND AND PICTURE YOURSELF VICTORIOUS

Visualize Your Success

As you visualize your success, I want you to form a mental template of how you want to look. This should not be a picture of someone else, a model, movie star, or celebrity. This should be a picture of a leaner, healthier, happier you. It might be helpful if you set aside a time and a place to visualize. What you are essentially doing is creating a mental picture of yourself having succeeded with weight loss. You are combining your body and your mind. Visualizing this success takes practice. I am not talking about daydreaming nor am I advocating self-absorption or overt narcissism. Rather, this is a personal self-assessment. Dr. JoAnn Dahlkoetter, author of *Your Performing Edge,* states, "Take the best you have been and the best you can possibly be and take a picture." You've heard the expression "a picture is worth a thousand words." That's what I am asking you to do— picture yourself victorious at weight loss. Think of this as a form of meditation. It can ultimately be relaxing and quite calming and take the stress *out* of weight loss.

Positive Reinforcement

A highly significant factor in my success rate with clients has always been based on continual motivation and positive reinforcement of their behavior. We all know how great it makes us feel to hear a boss, spouse, or partner say, "You're doing a great job." It motivates us to keep doing that great job and encourages us to try even harder. I continually instruct my staff on the benefits of positive reinforcement and urge them to provide it liberally to all clients. They need it. We all need it (especially children), yet unfortunately so few of us receive enough of it in our professional and private lives. Consequently, I don't want you to have to rely on one person or other individuals to provide this reassurance that you *will* succeed at losing the weight. I want you to use the technique of *visualization* to give yourself that motivation, encouragement, and positive reinforcement. I want you to begin developing that confidence from within.

Once Again, Go for the Internal Rather Than the External

You are going to use *internal* stimuli rather than external stimuli. Why? Because the internal is in *your* control. No one else can control what is inside of you. Sure, it will be great as you start losing weight and your friends and colleagues notice your progress and remark, "Gee, you really look different. What have you been doing?" But for right now, as you begin developing the belief in your ability to flip, there is nothing external for these people to see. Obviously, what they will first notice are the external changes that occur later, but you and I know that it is the internal motivation that comes from within you that is the driving force behind this external transformation. To help you keep that internal motivational level high, perform the following exercise: Begin by locating a full-length mirror in your home, ideally someplace that provides you with privacy. Take an objective look at your body in that mirror. For some readers, it may have been a long time since they *really* looked at themselves and evaluated their appearance. For years, I have heard men and women talk about how they cringe at the thought of buying a bathing suit. They were frightened at the thought of having to see themselves in a full-length mirror and face that reality. For some, it has prompted them to call me and say, "I just went bathing suit shopping and realized that I have to get a handle on my weight and appearance. Please call me so we can put a program

VISUALIZE THE FLIP

Take a Good Look at Your Body in a Mirror

together." Their visual image was the catalyst. Trust me, it works. While the visualization was external, it can inspire the motivation necessary to produce the internal flip of the switch.

Actually, this evaluation of yourself in a full-length mirror would be even more beneficial without clothing, but I will leave that decision to you. Regardless of what you are wearing or not wearing, I want you to take an inventory of your body. It's just you. Take your time. We rush through so many things in our lives, we ought to be able to find a few minutes to look at our most important asset, our body.

Next, I want you to take out a pen or pencil and fill in your response to the sentences in the space provided at right. Try to avoid the typical "I hate everything about my body." It's a shallow remark and comes from avoidance and being unwilling to try. You are dismissing your current body without even giving it a chance. I absolutely do not believe that you dislike *everything* about your body. Evaluate from top to bottom (no pun intended). Do you like your shoulders, chest, arms? Some people have a well-shaped body, but just too much of it. Start at the neck, then keep turning around and work your way down to your feet. I am positive that there is some aspect of your body that you like. It may even be that you have great skin, perfect toes, shapely ankles, graceful fingers, whatever. Just use this time to reintroduce yourself to what lives below the chin.

I had a professionally successful, attractive client who was a Slow Gainer. She never had a weight problem as a child, adolescent, or young adult, but in her thirties, she experienced the classic pattern of slow weight gain until finally she was fifty years old and twenty-five pounds heavier than she had been in her twenties. She used an expression to describe herself that has stayed with me and that I have shared with

EXERCISE 2

VISUALIZE THE FLIP
Body Description
I like this about my body:

_____

_____

_____

_____

_____

_____

I don't like this about my body:

_____

_____

_____

_____

_____

_____

many others. She called herself a "talking head." By this, she meant that she had been successful most of her adult life as a woman who used her mind, her brains, and her facility with language to get ahead. Everything came from the neck up. Now she wanted to put the two pieces together, the mind and the body. She wanted to complete the package and duplicate the success that she had achieved as a "talking head" with her body. This wasn't easy. It required developing a whole new way of looking at herself. It eventually worked, but believe me, it took some time.

Here's how we accomplished it. I asked her to evaluate her body in a full-length mirror. I then asked her to visualize what she would look and feel like with a thinner, more attractive body. I urged her to develop a picture in her mind (especially since she had been so successful using her mind in other areas of her life) to motivate her now to flip. Using this technique over and over, she gradually progressed. Each week she was better at visualizing a thinner version of herself, until she reached the point where her vision and the reality coincided.

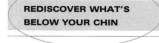

REDISCOVER WHAT'S
BELOW YOUR CHIN

Joanne Wears a Size 8

I have one more story that relates to this visual issue. In November 2000, I did a program with ABC's *Good Morning America* called "Lock the Door, Lose the Weight." We locked seven overweight people in a house on the north shore of Chicago and provided them with a nutritionist, a psychologist, a chef, and me. We monitored their progress for one month and then continued monitoring them throughout the following year. One of the most successful participants, Joanne, a forty-something new mom, has lost more than forty pounds to date and looks great. She continues to monitor her caloric intake and always does the strength and resistance exercises I prescribed for her. This past Christmas, she said that she was opening presents that were all size 8. She said she had a "right, like I can wear a size 8" look on her face. She had spent the last few years between a size 12 and 14. Guess what? She fit in every size 8. She was shocked. Joanne *can* fit into a size 8! Obviously, her family members visualized her as a size 8, but she didn't. She needed to *see* it to believe it. Had she participated in the visualization exercise, she would have been able to readily accept her new size. Joanne can fit into a size 8. By the way, now she's pushing for a size 6 and visualizes herself at that size.

Pick the Private Rather Than the Public Setting

One more important point about looking in the mirror: If you plan on going to a health club or gym to exercise, odds are that you are going to have to look at yourself in a mirror. You'll end up seeing yourself in the mirror from every conceivable angle. There is no getting around it. For some of you, this may be a difficult experience. Why not have that first experience in the privacy of your home rather than in a public setting? That way, you will be better prepared for the mirror and any emotions that may surface.

So, take that long, detailed inventory of your body. Consider this part of the research data as you begin to visualize a "new," thinner you. Then proceed to the next exercise.

For this next exercise, I want you to go back in time. I want you to find old pictures of yourself in which you liked the way you looked. I know what some of you are saying—"I have never, ever liked the way I looked"—but I don't believe it. I am trying to get you past the negative relationship you have with your body. Each and every one of us, at some point in time, has seen a picture of ourselves that we liked. Quite possibly you were not at what you would consider your "ideal weight," but I am sure, at some point in your past, you felt you looked healthier and thinner than you do now. That's the photo I want you to locate. For many of you this may be a wedding picture or a photo at an important event or time in your life. That was *you,* the person in the photograph was *you.* I have to repeat, that was *you.* You undoubtedly held on to this photo because you did like the way

EXERCISE 3

VISUALIZE THE FLIP
Find Old Pictures

you looked. Look at it and, more important, recalling the previous chapter, believe it. Absorb that visual. You looked that way once, you can look that way again. That photo represents what was once your reality and you can make it your reality once again.

I do this all the time with clients. Often, at the initial interview, I look around their home or office, identify a picture that clearly reflects a thinner, healthier time in their lives, and ask them about it. Keep in mind, people rarely display unflattering pictures of themselves. I will often say, "How old were you in this picture?" or "Were you exercising when this shot was taken?" Anything to give me some additional information as to what has changed between the photo and the present.

I want you to attach this picture to the space provided below and, just as I instructed you in exercise 4 in the previous chapter, write down next to the picture what you were doing with regard to eating, activity, and exercise at the time the photo was taken and the present. For example: "At the time this photo was taken on _____, I was doing the following with regard to eating and exercise."

YOU WERE THIS SIZE
ONCE BEFORE, AND YOU
WILL BE AGAIN

Your next exercise is to determine what has changed from the time this photo was taken and now. To do so, I want you to write in the space provided at right what transpired between the time this photo was taken and now.

Here are some of the comments I have heard from clients over the years:

- "When I was thirty, I lived in New York City and walked home from work every day. I was really busy and had to force myself to do it sometimes, but three to four days out of every week, I walked thirty blocks home. Once we moved to the suburbs, I was forced to drive everywhere."

- "When I lived in Detroit, there was a gym about a mile from my home. Three times a week, I would leave the kids with my husband and go to the club religiously. Then we moved and I never got around to finding a gym nearby."

- "Before I got promoted, I never had a problem managing my weight. Then the business travel and entertainment started, and it has never been the same."

- "I gained forty-five pounds with the baby. The first twenty came off quickly. Then I struggled with the final twenty-five and have actually never gotten them off. I feel like the baby just ruined my body. I am convinced my body will never be the same."

Each of these comments demonstrates that some sort of change occurred between the photo and now. Here is what transpired. Exercise/activity diminished, eating increased, time became an issue, or you simply

VISUALIZE THE FLIP

Determine What Has Changed

Between the time this photo was taken and now, the following has changed:

VISUALIZE THE FLIP

**Get Out Your Old Clothes—
Seeing Is Believing**

got away from the belief that you could maintain your weight. Review your comments associated with the photo. Any conclusions? Think about what enabled you to be happier with your weight in the past, then apply some of those same principles to your situation today.

You have now done an analysis of your present body. You have identified old photographs that provided you with a visual that you liked, and you analyzed what you were doing with regard to exercise, eating, and attitude at the time of the photo. Here is the final exercise of the chapter: Every month I want you to go to your closet, attic, or wherever you store old clothing you no longer wear. Take out the pieces that are too small for you and realize a simple fact: You once fit into these clothes. They were your reality. These clothes, just like the photos of the old, leaner you, are proof that you once weighed less. Remember my client who could no longer fit into her favorite cashmere coat? She had actually forgotten that she once fit into it. The old adage "Seeing is believing" definitely applies. Seeing a coat that she once fit into was for her the catalyst—it was her visual.

How Many Sizes Can You Wear?

Some clients have told me that they have complete wardrobes sitting in the back of their closets, in another room, or in the attic that they can no longer fit into. I urged them to get some of these clothes out, or at least their favorites, and I want you to do the same. Take a suit, a dress, or a pair of jeans, something that you really liked, and hang it on the outside of your closet or in plain view to remind you that you once fit into these clothes. Hold the suit, dress, or pair of jeans up to your body, close your eyes, and remember what it felt like to fit into this piece of clothing. Then, hold it away from you and look at it. This represents your past shape, a size that you liked. Now, visualize what you will look like wearing it again. Keep that picture in your mind, believe you can achieve it, and turn that mental picture into a reality.

Let's explore this a little further. Why have you held on to these clothes in the first place? It's quite obvious. You kept the garment because you held on to the dream that you could once again wear it. My goal is to turn that dream into a reality. Yes, it does take time, effort, and dedication. But, just for a moment, visualize what you will look and feel like when you can open your closet and pick out anything—I mean anything—that you like, put it on, and feel great!

The Skinny Skirt

Diane Sawyer, one of my most successful clients to date, lost more than twenty-five pounds with my program. I remember the day she interviewed Janet Jackson and rushed home for our workout. In the past, she spoke of a "skinny skirt" that she loved and hoped to get back into. She actually kept it hanging in her *Good Morning America/PrimeTime* dressing room as a reminder. That day, as I rarely saw her in "work clothes," I commented on how great and thin she looked. She pointed down and said, "This is the skinny skirt. This is it!" Guess what? It fit perfectly. This visual tool had inspired her not to lose sight of her goal and kept her believing in her ability to stay flipped.

Visualize Yourself Stress Free

A recent study in the *Journal of Consulting and Clinical Psychology* reports that "researchers have found that simple self-hypnosis techniques (such as picturing yourself near a calm place like the ocean) can protect your immune system from the negative effects of acute stress." As you will learn in subsequent chapters, stress can subject your body to a myriad of negative effects, including anxiety, overeating, increased production of the hormone cortisol (which leads you

LOSE THE STRESS AND
YOU'LL LOSE THE WEIGHT

to become overweight; see pages 89–90 in Chapter 4), fatigue, and sleep deprivation. Use calming visualization to reduce stress, which will enable you to lose weight.

Take a moment. Close your eyes. Visualize what you will look like ten, twenty, thirty, or more pounds lighter. Really picture yourself. Really see it. Reread the first chapter and *believe* it can happen. Find your own "skinny skirt." Visualize what you will look like and feel like when you can once again wear that piece of clothing. You are visualizing success.

EVENTUALLY THE
ZIPPER WILL ZIP

PUTTING IT ALL TOGETHER TO FLIP

You now understand the powerful effects of visualization. You are going to begin linking your mind with your body. From Chapter 1, you are starting to *believe* you can flip. Now, you can create a mental template in your mind of a thinner, healthier, happier you. To further this process, I have asked you to do the following:

• Complete an inventory of your present body's appearance.

• Identify old photographs of yourself that you like and document what you were doing with regard to eating, exercise, and activity at the time the photo was taken.

• Select old clothing that you want to once again wear and visualize it on your body.

The purpose of these three exercises was to demonstrate to you that you once weighed less than you do now. Stop doubting that you can be at that weight again. You have the data to prove you can. You will lose weight. You need to frequently revisit these three techniques. Remember what I told you in Chapter 1? There are certain exercises that you must agree to perform *each* month. Therefore, at the first of the month, look at your body, study old photos, and by all means, start to try on the old clothes. I know in the beginning they won't fit, but you will eventually see the buttons getting closer or the zipper beginning to zip. This *is* thrilling and motivating. It indicates that you are on your way. Also, doing this only once a month allows your body to significantly change, which will prove even more motivating. To enable you to keep this monthly inventory, you'll find a year's worth of worksheets, including a place where you can note your weight (see page 284 for weighing guidelines), at the end of this book, one for each month, plus a blank one that you can photocopy to continue your inventory beyond one year (which I highly recommend).

The novelist Thomas Wolfe (*Look Homeward Angel*) popularized the phrase "You can't go home again." Well, maybe you can't go home again, but you can return to a size and shape that you were when you lived in that home.

In Part 1, "It Can Happen to You," you were presented with a series of mental exercises to assist you in beginning to flip the switch. In the next part, "What's Kept You from Flipping?" I will investigate and help you to navigate the most common excuses I have heard over the years that have prevented many individuals from flipping. I will not allow you to sabotage yourself. Ready? Let's take those excuses one by one and overcome them.

3 "I Don't Have the Time"

I was recently conducting a weight-management workshop for new mothers. These women had previously been in good shape, exercised regularly, and watched their diets. Now, with an infant, their time no longer seemed to be within their control. The additional responsibility of the baby, plus a job for some, on top of their already full schedule, left little extra time for them to focus on themselves. Each and every new mom, in her own words, repeated a similar phrase: "My time is no longer mine," or "I don't have a moment to spare," or "I can't seem to get anything done." After an hour, I asked the class a simple question: "Why is your time no longer within your control? Who is taking this control away from you?" Most said, "Why, the baby, of course." To which I replied, "No, it isn't the baby, it's *you*.

"First of all, raise your hand if there is someone at home on the weekends to help you with the baby," I said. All but one new mom raised her hand. "Okay, why can't this person watch the baby for thirty or forty minutes on both Saturday and Sunday while you exercise?" All heads tilted to the side as they thought about it. Then came the nods. Presto, they just created the time for two workout sessions a week. Many times, the solution can be as easy as this.

One of the most frequent excuses put forth by individuals to rationalize their inability to flip the switch is lack of time. "Oh yes," they say, "I truly want to flip. I'm ready to flip. But I just don't have the time." Yes, time is a finite commodity, but it can be managed to enable you to succeed at weight loss and structure your life more efficiently. In this chapter, you will learn to make time your ally. It no longer will be your enemy. I want you to look at the time you spend on yourself as one of the most valuable things in your life. Right now, you are making time for some combination of your work, spouse, kids, home, holidays, volunteering, and so on, in addition to probably hundreds of other tasks. Now I want you to put *yourself* high up on that list and make the time required to flip your highest

> "THE SECRET OF GETTING AHEAD IS GETTING STARTED."
> —SALLY BERGER

"I DON'T HAVE THE TIME"

**Construct a Time-Log Journal—
Create Awareness**

6 A.M. _____

7 A.M. _____

8 A.M. _____

9 A.M. _____

10 A.M. _____

11 A.M. _____

12 A.M. _____

1 P.M. _____

2 P.M. _____

3 P.M. _____

4 P.M. _____

5 P.M. _____

6 P.M. _____

7 P.M _____

8 P.M. _____

9 P.M. _____

10 P.M. _____

11 P.M. _____

priority. This is not being selfish. On the contrary, this is about being smart and taking control of your *body* and your *mind*. I know you can do it.

Start with the Basics

Let's start with the basics of time management and determine how much time is actually available to you on a daily basis. Given that there are twenty-four hours a day, and that the average American sleeps approximately seven of those hours, that leaves seventeen hours available each day for everything else. Therefore, given a seven-day week, a total of 119 hours are available on a weekly basis.

**7 DAYS × 17 HOURS = 119 HOURS AVAILABLE
ON A WEEKLY BASIS**

And by the way:

**119 HOURS × 60 MINUTES = 7,140 MINUTES AVAILABLE
ON A WEEKLY BASIS**

Think about that: You have 119 hours or 7,140 minutes a week to accomplish all that you set out to achieve. That's a considerable amount of time. Visualize what you can accomplish. With that in mind, begin the first exercise of this chapter at left. The purpose of this journal (in addition to the other journals I am asking you to construct in this book) is to create behavior awareness. Frequently we are unaware of how we use our time, just as we are often unaware of how we spend our money (see Chapter 5) and what we eat (see Chapter 7). I encourage you to be brutally honest as you construct this journal. No one is going to see this journal but you. Recall what I said in the preceding chapter: Seeing is believing. Documenting how you use your time will enable you to find the time to flip. For the first week, I want you to record every activity you perform each day and the time required to perform that activity. If you watch a soap, put it in. If you nap, gossip, talk on the phone, put it in. Record every activity in your time-log journal. This is similar to what I will ask you to do in Chapter 7, "'I Love to Eat,'" where I instruct you to keep a food diary. While the food journal is a long-range exercise, you only need to complete this time log for one week. One week will provide you with the information you require. Remember, we are striving to create behavior awareness with this exercise.

On the right, I give you an example of a typical weekday in my time-log journal. If you examine my day closely, you will notice that I'm exercising in the early afternoon. I find that it gives me a jump start for the rest of the day. Without it, I oftentimes feel sluggish. I recommend this option to clients who have exercise rooms at their office, at their office building, or at a nearby health club/gym. While this option may be somewhat easier for men than for women, don't be concerned because once you see the style of exercise I prescribe in Chapter 8, "'I Hate to Exercise,'" you will see that the routines I've created do not necessarily cause you to perspire profusely. Hair and makeup damage is minimal and you may not feel the need to shower.

My time log represents an average Monday through Thursday when I am in New York City working with clients, and I'll be the first to admit I have a tight schedule. In Chicago, my Fridays consist primarily of office administration and writing. Also on Fridays, I take my daughter to school, exercise in the morning, and then go to my office. Weekend schedules are different. I spend time with my wife and children (I seem to attend a zillion kids' birthday

JIM KARAS'S WEEKDAY TIME-LOG JOURNAL

Time	Activity
6:30–7:00	Wake up, eat breakfast, get dressed
7:00–8:00	Return phone calls and e-mail and scan various newspapers
8:00	Depart for first client
8:30–9:30	Client session
9:45–10:45	Client session
11:00–12:00	Client session
12:00–12:15	Lunch, usually at a salad bar or deli counter
12:30–1:30	Client session
1:45–2:45	**Exercise**
3:00–4:00	Client session
4:00–4:45	Return phone calls and e-mail
5:00–6:00	Client session
6:15–7:15	Client session
7:30–8:00	Dinner at home
8:00–10:00	Combination watching television, reading, writing, or returning phone calls and e-mail or out to dinner
10:00–10:15	Bed, possibly a little reading, sleep

JIM KARAS'S WEEKEND TIME-LOG JOURNAL

7:00–7:30	Get up and play with the kids
7:30–8:00	Breakfast with the family
8:00–8:30	Return phone calls and e-mail
8:30–9:30	My wife exercises and I watch the kids
9:30–10:30	My turn to **exercise** while my wife watches the kids
10:30–11:00	Shower and dress
11:00	Depart for the office
11:10–3:00	Work in the office (kids sometimes come to the office with me)
3:15–5:30	Play with the kids, go shopping, sleep (I love to nap), read, or watch television
5:30	Either help with dinner at home or get ready to go out

parties), visit with friends, and write. On the left is a typical weekend morning/afternoon schedule. I follow this schedule almost every Saturday and Sunday. It's a great way to guarantee that I get at least two workouts in each week. It's also a nice way for me to have time alone with my children, which I greatly enjoy.

The Goal is Three Sessions a Week

Notice that in my two time-log examples, I have included an exercise session each day. The reality is that I don't always work out every day of the week; however, I always manage to get in a minimum of three sessions a week. It all depends on my travel schedule, which typically consists of client sessions, workshops, and speaking engagements. I urge you to schedule at least one additional exercise session each week than you will realistically have time for. In other words, *overschedule those sessions.* That way, if a situation arises that prevents you from making one session, by week's end you will still have accomplished your goal of working out three times.

Note that I have scheduled one-hour workouts. This is not always the case. Sometimes, I do a quick twenty- or thirty-minute intense workout if that is all that my time will allow. In Chapter 8, "'I Hate to Exercise,'" I will explain to you how you can get a great deal accomplished in a minimal amount of time.

As I am writing this book, my wife is not working. She is taking time off from her career to be with the kids. Since her schedule is probably similar to that of many stay-at-home moms with young children, I have included her weekday time-log journal as an illustration (see opposite page).

Ellen's plan is to exercise in the mornings. This may

be the only time of the day that she has a chance to get it accomplished. She also exercises in our home while the baby is sleeping. This is something I often recommend to stay-at-home moms. That is why two of my three exercise programs in Chapter 8 can be performed in a home setting.

Both my wife and I, one of us working outside the home and one of us working inside the home, have managed to schedule exercise into our daily routines. Just like me, Ellen exercises three to four times each week. Again, planning is the key. (Remember, my first book was titled *The Business **Plan** for the Body*.) Nearly everyone's daily schedule requires some planning and the making of choices. I am asking you to decide to improve yourself emotionally and physically. There is nothing selfish about this decision of focusing on yourself and finding time for exercise. In fact, a healthier, more productive you will better contribute to the lives of others. Repeat after me: **"Taking time for myself is not selfish."** Quite the contrary, it's smart. You will be healthier, happier, more patient, less anxious, and leaner. How could anyone possibly object to you taking the time to achieve that goal? Construct your time-log journal and continue reading.

Are You Finding the Time?

Okay, how is your time-log journal shaping up? Are you starting to see time where you may be able to fit exercise into your schedule? Is it possible you can delete something from your present schedule or reduce the time spent on other activities to carve out time to exercise? Remember, time management is about choices and the setting of priorities. The fact that you are reading this book clearly indicates that you created time for yourself. The same will happen

ELLEN KARAS'S WEEKDAY TIME-LOG JOURNAL

6:00–7:00	Our toddler, Evan, gets up
7:00–8:00	Olivia, our five-and-a-half-year-old, gets up; breakfast; get everyone dressed and ready to leave for school
8:00–8:45	Drop Olivia off at school and return home
9:00	Put Evan down for his nap
9:15–10:15	**Exercise in the apartment with SPRI tubing, Resist-A-Ball, and free weights (see Chapter 8 for more details)**
10:30	Evan gets up
10:15–11:00	Shower, get dressed, plan for the day
11:15	Pick up Olivia at school
11:45–12:30	Return home for lunch with the kids
12:30–2:00	Take children to classes or play dates
2:00–5:00	Shop, clean, cook, and monitor the kids
5:00–6:00	Prepare and eat dinner
6:00–7:00	Children's baths and ready for bed
7:00–7:20	Evan to bed
7:20–7:40	Stories for Olivia and tuck her in
7:45	Collapse

with exercise. Read through the following options to assist you with your exercise scheduling.

Explore the Exercise-Time Options

Workout Time—Option 1:
First Thing in the Morning

For many individuals, if exercise doesn't take place first thing in the morning, it's not going to happen. Why? For a lot of people, early morning is the *only* option because of their schedule. For working men and women, if they exercise at, say, 6:00 or 6:30 A.M., they can get dressed and be at their jobs by 8:00 or 8:30, depending on commute time. This option provides a great advantage. One only needs to shower and get dressed once each day, which saves considerable time, especially in comparison to exercising later in the day, when you most likely will change and shower a second time. For stay-at-home parents, morning may also be the time when the kids are still sleeping, which enables the parents to concentrate and exercise without distraction.

Over the years, my weight-loss management firm in Chicago, Jim Karas Personal Training, LLC, has experienced an increased demand for the 5:30, 6:00, and 6:30 A.M. time slots. Numerous case studies also indicate that those who plan to exercise first thing in the morning have the greatest likelihood of following through. That's because later in the day, situations can arise that many times will prevent you from exercising. These situations place demands on your time and can make you feel guilty about allocating time for yourself. So think about it—does first thing in the morning make sense for you? Try it. You may be surprised to find that the early-morning boost really gets both your physical and your mental juices flowing.

Workout Time—Option 2:
Early Midmorning

This option seems to work best for stay-at-home parents with young children, those with very flexible hours, retirees, and seniors. At my daughter's school, more than half of the parents are wearing exercise clothes when they drop off their kids (see my opening anecdote for the next chapter). They go directly to the gym, an exercise class, or back home to exercise. This is a great time slot if one has young children. The kids get up so early that most parents don't have an opportunity to exercise in the early morning. But once the kids are out of the house, this is your "window" of opportunity. Use it. If you exercise between 8:30 and 10:00 A.M., you then have the time to get cleaned up and ready for the day, and as with the very-early-morning option, you only need to shower and dress once, a major time-saver for everyone.

For those people who don't have children at home and perhaps fall into the retiree or senior category, this option can also be very effective. After a leisurely breakfast and reading the paper, they exercise and then carry on with the rest of their day. For workers who have flexible schedules and go to work later in the day, midmorning is also a perfect time.

IF YOU'RE "STUCK" AT HOME, YOU CAN DO MY WORKOUT *AT HOME*

Workout Time—Option 3:
Lunchtime Workout

You may have guessed that this time option is my personal favorite. I love the boost a lunchtime workout gives me for the rest of the afternoon. Lots of working men and women prefer this option and fit it into their schedules on a weekly basis. For many of us, an hour is all we can devote to our lunch break, so the key to a successful lunchtime workout is the proximity of the workout facility. If you don't have equipment in your office or office building, locate a workout facility that is close by. That way, a thirty- to forty-minute exercise session is possible, which will allow enough time to shower, grab a light lunch, and return to the office. Tight time frame, but it does work.

An added benefit of exercising at this time is that you will find that you eat less at lunch. Why? Basically for two reasons. First, after a workout, you generally feel physically lean and energized. The thought of putting heavy food in your stomach is unappealing. Second, mentally you feel accomplished after completing a workout and want to complement that feeling by eating a lighter lunch. Consequently, you tend to eat less. For those people who eat lunch right after a workout, I recommend options such as a turkey sandwich with lettuce, tomato, and Dijon mustard. Another good choice is a salad or yogurt. Foods like these can easily be prepared in advance at home or purchased at a deli, grocery store, or convenience mart, thus eliminating the *time* a meal in a sit-down restaurant entails.

Give it a try. You may find that lunchtime is your best exercise option. Remember, you are not exercising every day, so some days you can have a regular sit-down lunch with your friends or business associates.

Workout Time—Option 4:
Early Evening

Many of us need to be at work as early as possible; often the demands of the office, home, and children are just too much to allow us to take time for ourselves during daytime hours. But either right before or soon after dinner, many have found that they can carve out the time to exercise. Both men and women, either working or not, may find that at 5:00, 6:00, or 7:00 P.M., they can get in thirty to forty minutes of exercise. They may be tired and stressed out from the day, but this can be the perfect time to blow off a little steam, think, process the events of the day, and set up for a relaxing evening.

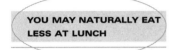

YOU MAY NATURALLY EAT
LESS AT LUNCH

Like a lunchtime workout, an end-of-the-day workout may also give you a boost that keeps you alert and helps you to stay productive in the evening. My weight-loss management firm has many couples who exercise together at the end of the day. They find that it is a great way to spend time together, talk about their day, and take care of their bodies at the same time. It works. Or, if the kids are little, it may make sense to do what my wife and I do on the weekends (note: I said *weekends,* not weekdays). One parent gets to exercise first, while the other deals with the children, then you switch. Everyone gets to exercise, the kids aren't left alone, and the job gets done.

If you do select early evening but want to exercise after dinner, I'd recommend you eat half your meal at dinnertime and the other half after your exercise session. This way, you won't feel full and uncomfortable when you exercise. It also will provide you with additional energy for the workout.

It's important to keep the meals relatively simple. I recommend some protein, such as lean meat, white meat turkey/chicken without the skin, or fish. Add to that a small salad or steamed vegetables. When you eat a heavy meal or mix many different types of foods, your stomach has to work harder to digest the food (I will address this issue in the next chapter). That depletes energy. So keep it small and simple before the workout and plan on eating another small meal later in the evening. If you don't eat dinner, make sure to eat a healthy snack such as ½ cup of low-fat yogurt, ½ cup of low-fat cottage cheese, a piece of fruit, or a piece of toast (60- or 70-calorie bread, please).

Workout Time—Option 5:
Late-Evening Exercise

Though the following option is not used by many, it does work for some, especially "night" people. For those who find that they have more energy in the late-evening hours than they do during the day, this is the best option. There are also individuals for whom an exercise session is not possible unless it takes place during the late evening. For whatever reason, time simply is not available in their schedule to exercise at any other time. Once the children are in bed or they are finally home from work, they find they *do* have the time to devote to exercise. My weight-loss management firm has a number of physicians who exercise at this time because surgery, rounds, or being on call does not allow for exercise at other times during the day.

Note that a couple of concerns should be addressed with regard to this option: First, as in the early-evening example, be careful with what you eat for dinner. Second, keep in mind that exercise does tend to overly stimulate some individuals and makes it difficult for them to relax and sleep after exercise. *Consumer Reports on Health* states that "exercise promotes wakefulness by causing the release of nerve-stimulating hormones and elevating the body's core temperature, so it's hard to fall asleep soon after working out. But, the more energy you expend at any time during the day or night, the sleepier you'll be at bedtime and possibly the better you'll sleep." So, if you do try this option and find it difficult to fall asleep, then considering one of the other options is probably a better choice. But I do know some people who benefit from late-evening exercise when it's time to fall asleep. They say that the exercise relieves the stress of the day and allows them to sleep peacefully.

Workout Time—Option 6:
Short Bouts of Exercise

Recent case studies have demonstrated that short bouts of exercise at various times of the day are just as effective as one thirty-minute or longer exercise session. If a ten-minute session two or three times a day works best with your schedule, then plan on it. Plan to exercise first thing in the morning for ten minutes, then once again before or after lunch and then finally the last ten-minute session in the evening. And remember, my suggested exercise routine will normally not make you perspire profusely and need to shower afterward. You may be able to close your office door, perform three or four exercises in about ten minutes, then resume work. Or perhaps while watching your favorite television show, you can perform a few exercises during the commercials. Or turn your "coffee" break into a ten-minute exercise break. The choice is yours. Just know that you can exercise for brief periods of time throughout the day if that's the most effective way to keep you consistent and still produce dramatic results.

TURN YOUR COFFEE
BREAK INTO AN
EXERCISE BREAK

Finally, I'd like to call your attention to recent research that supports the benefits of short bouts of exercise performed at home. A study reported in the *Journal of the American Medical Association* separated 148 sedentary women into three groups. The first group performed a traditional one-hour exercise session, the second did multiple short bouts of exercise in a health club or gym, and the third did multiple short bouts of exercise with home exercise equipment. At the end of the eighteen-month program, weight loss was significantly greater in the third group who performed short bouts of exercise in the home. The researchers concluded that "access to home exercise equipment facilitated adherence to the exercise program and may thus explain this group's improvement in long-term weight loss." So keep in mind, the more convenient the location of the exercise equipment, the more apt you are to use it.

GO "SHORT" AT WORK OR AT HOME

Don't Suffer from Decision Dilemma

What about those individuals whose schedules allow them to exercise at *any* time during the day? These are lucky people. For them, a brief cautionary note: Consistency is the key. Having too much time can create "decision dilemma." When presented with too many options, some people end up floundering and no exercise session actually occurs. Pick a workout time that fits your lifestyle and stick with it!

I have heard from clients, women in particular, who state that they get up and put exercise clothing on in anticipation that they will exercise at some point. However, an actual session time is never established. These individuals spend the whole day hoping to exercise, but never act on that hope. They think by wearing the exercise clothing, the exercise will automatically take place. This is somewhat akin to buying this book. Not only do you have to buy it, you then have to read it and act upon it. Please be aware of this trap.

WEARING EXERCISE CLOTHING DOES NOT CONSTITUTE A "WORKOUT"

Don't Overlook Your Biological Rhythms

In selecting an exercise time that is best for you, consider your needs and personality. If you had the option of exercising whenever you want, what would be the best time for you? You know yourself better than anyone. Numerous studies have long noted that various individuals learn better at certain times of the day, are more alert during certain times of the day, are more productive during certain times of the day. Think about how all of this relates to you.

Don't Forget to Consider Where You Are Going to Exercise

If you like the energy you derive from a busy health club or gym, then by all means go there during prime-time hours (weekdays between 6:00 and 9:00 A.M. or 5:00 and 8:00 P.M.). If you would prefer a more relaxed environment, with easier access to the equipment, then go during off-peak time. If you have identified a television program you like to watch or listen to while exercising, then do it during that time. That way, you get to enjoy the program and exercise simultaneously, which can help to keep you more consistent and motivated.

Ease Yourself into Exercise

The goal is to select the time and place that work for you. If you feel comfortable with it, you will be better able to incorporate exercise into your daily routine. You will also exercise more efficiently and derive more from the time you invest. Experiment. Try exercising at different times to determine the option best suited to you. It doesn't matter where or when you exercise. What does matter is that you create time in your schedule to do so.

So, complete your time log for one week. Then review all the workout time options I describe. As you do this, keep one point in mind: If you presently are not exercising, then strive to perform one session a week. Make a deal with yourself and decide, for the next four weeks, to fit one exercise session in each week. Then after you have achieved that goal on a regular basis, add another session for the next four-week period. Eventually, as you'll see in Chapter 8, you'll work up to three times a week. The key is to ease yourself into the program rather than set unrealistic expectations and fail.

SELECT A TIME AND PLACE THAT WORK FOR YOU AND BE CONSISTENT

Avoiding a feeling of failure is crucial to your success. Most of you have been through this routine. You woke up one day and said, "I am going to totally change how I eat and exercise starting today!" Did you purchase exercise equipment? Perhaps. Did you make a New Year's resolution? Probably. Did it work? *Did you flip?* No? What happened? You resolved to undertake the difficult task of weight loss, made an announcement, and believed that—*shazam!*—it would all fall into place. Unfortunately, it doesn't work that way. Actually, very few goals in life are that easily attained. Weight loss is a complicated process leading to a physical change. In addition, it's also a mental process. So that you don't fall into the same old traps, I am going to help you to establish realistic physical and mental goals.

Thirty to Forty Minutes Gets the Job Done

Exercising about thirty to forty minutes once a week for the next four weeks is realistic. One session (or thirty to forty minutes of exercise in short bouts) a week may not sound like much, but if you haven't been exercising, that time to exercise represents a significant departure from your current lifestyle. Ease yourself into the program and then progress. After the first four weeks, add a second session or another thirty to forty minutes in short bouts and continue to exercise twice weekly for the next four weeks. When you reach the point where you can perform three exercise sessions a week on a regular basis, then you have reached the "flip the switch" magic number. I'll explain why that's the case in detail in Chapter 8, "'I Hate to Exercise.'" But for now, trust me, three times a week gets the job done.

Thirty to forty minutes is all the time that is required if you exercise intelligently and consistently, and employ the right exercise prescription to meet your goals. Once again, we will discuss these factors in Chapter 8—including the proper and most effective ways to exercise—in detail, but for now, realize that a thirty- to forty-minute exercise session is enormously beneficial and not just for beginners but for all individuals.

Make Time for the Right Food Choices

Fitting exercise into your weekly schedule is your first time-management assignment. Now you'll learn to find the time to plan

"I DON'T HAVE THE TIME"

Determine Which Meals Will Be Eaten at Home and Which Meals Will Be Eaten Out

the right food choices. This will be easier. Start by looking at your schedule for the coming week and map out your eating plan with the help of exercise 2. This exercise requires a minimal amount of time. Once again, the key is planning. Leave little to chance. Look at your work schedule, if applicable, and your personal schedule. What events, dates, or meetings that include food do you see on the horizon for the coming week? Start with today and project forward. Do not overlook any meal—breakfast, lunch, dinner, or even just a snack. All should be noted at left.

As you review your week, determine how you can effectively manage these situations or events from an eating standpoint. Ask yourself how many of these meals are within your control. If this is a business breakfast, lunch, or dinner, do you have any input as to where these meals will take place and what foods will be served? If so, choose the restaurants or order those foods for the office meeting that you know will keep the calories down. If this is an office breakfast meeting, add some low-calorie yogurt or fruit to the typical Danish, doughnut, muffin, bagel fare. If you're not in charge of the food, politely approach the individual who will place the order and request some low-calorie alternatives. Rarely will anyone object. On the contrary, you might be surprised to hear the person say, "I noticed you are looking so much better. Is this what you are doing? Tell me what you're eating." You'll also probably notice that a lot of your colleagues will select yogurt or fruit if it's offered. Or, if you can't effect a change, eat at home and have some coffee, tea, or water at the meeting.

This sort of planning does not require much time. Just take a moment and think. Clearly, lunch or dinner with friends will be much more in your control than a preplanned business event. The important thing is to try to make the best of each situation and to keep in mind that you are ultimately the one in control of what you put in your mouth no matter the menu or the venue.

Scope Out Restaurants

For a restaurant meal, call the restaurant in advance and ask them to fax the menu to your home or office. If that's not possible, discuss the menu with the restaurant personnel on the phone for a few minutes. I do this for clients all the time. That way, if someone wants to go to a new restaurant or one you haven't previously visited, you will know beforehand what's on the menu and determine if this is a "good" place for you. If it isn't good for you foodwise, at least you can make the best of the situation. I want you to eliminate the unexpected where food is concerned. Seeing the menu in advance will also help with your food selection once you are in the restaurant because many times it's easy to become distracted with conversation and the activity in the restaurant. You also don't want to keep others waiting and consequently make a quick selection that is fatal to your weight-loss plan. You retain control and save time by advance planning. In addition, each time you get another menu, keep it in a file at your home or office so that you have a place to turn when someone wants to select a restaurant. This will not only save you *time* in the future, which is what this chapter is helping you to accomplish, but also keep your eating program from experiencing an unforeseen setback.

Now consider those meals you will be eating at home or ordering in. If you are going to stop for carryout on the way home from the office or after having picked up the kids, then decide in advance where you will purchase it. Keep a file of carryout menus that will help you make this decision. A few minutes of planning takes most of the "unknown" out of the decision-making process and it lessens impulse purchases. You take a few minutes, and you save yourself hundreds, possibly thousands, of calories and *time*. A small investment in time and planning will yield great results when it comes to your food choices and ultimately your success at weight loss.

LEAVE THE KIDS AT HOME—AND EAT *BEFORE* YOU GO

Try not to bring the kids to the store. Nothing distracts you more than having a child who is tired, bored, and seduced by advertising begging for certain "treats" when you are trying to concentrate and get out of the store as soon as possible. Why do you think all the candy and toys are placed, along with the tabloids, directly at the checkout line? Those companies actually pay for that placement since it is so profitable. Even when you are alone, skip the peanut M&M's and just read the tabloids to find out which celebrity was recently abducted by aliens. You cannot lose your focus while in the store. Eliminate the distractions and, by planning, keep your focus. And, of course, never go to the grocery store hungry. Plan to have eaten beforehand or at least schedule a snack prior to shopping.

AVOID SUPERMARKET
SEDUCTION AND STICK
TO YOUR LIST

Fine-tune Your Supermarket Strategy

Of course, you do have much control over meals you prepare at home yourself. But here again, advance planning is the key to saving time and keeping your weight-loss strategy on course. Prior to going to your local supermarket, create a shopping list (I have done this for you in Chapter 7). Supermarkets are physically arranged to separate consumers from their money. Never forget this. Be aware that you will be tempted to deviate from your list when you first enter the store.

Supermarkets have invested large amounts of time, research, and money creating seductive food displays. As you begin your trek through this dangerous "commercial calorie zone," your power to resist is at its lowest. Why is this the case? Well, initially you have few items in your cart or basket. Bam! Immediately you encounter a high-profit item such as candy, cookies, or a high-calorie snack or prepared food and your thinking goes something like this: "I know it's not on my list. I haven't bought much yet. It doesn't require any preparation. It looks good." And in an instant it's in your shopping cart. It's not until you're in the checkout lane or unpacking your groceries at home that you become aware of what you bought or overbought. (We will talk about this in Chapter 5, "'I Don't Have the Money.'")

There's just one more rule to follow if you want to control the calories in your shopping cart: Stick to your list when you go through the store. Here's another idea: Several people have told me that they are eating so much healthier and have cut calories and food costs simply by using an Internet grocery shopper or ordering groceries by phone. Temptation and impulse are eliminated by using those kinds of services. Plus, you save a considerable amount of *time.* In some cities, you can also have a standard order that your grocery store will deliver each week. It may be boring to shop this way, but never underestimate the contribution food management plays in your success at weight loss. Again, it's all in the advance planning.

Become the Master of Your Time

When you began this chapter, you kept saying "I don't have the time to devote to weight loss. I'm too busy. I can't fit another thing into my schedule." Now you realize that you *are* the master of your time. You became the master of your time by planning. You do have time, kids or no kids, young or old, working or nonworking. I have shown you that successful weight loss does not have to entail a huge amount of time. What it does require is intelligent planning.

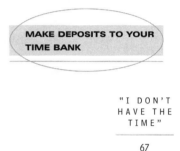

Consider the time *saved* as your weight loss improves your health. You are less apt to miss time at work, and when you're at work you'll undoubtedly be more productive and mentally alert. By dealing with fewer of these factors, you will actually *add* to your "time bank"— fewer deductions and more "time" deposits. In no time, you will see and feel an overwhelming difference in your body and, as you will read in the next chapter, you'll experience a dramatic increase in energy.

PUTTING IT ALL TOGETHER TO FLIP

- *Planning* is the key to weight management. *Plan when* you are going to exercise. *Plan what, when, and where* you are going to eat. Strategize.

- Time is within *your* control: You are the architect of your time.

- There are approximately 119 hours or 7,140 minutes available to you each week.

- Management of those 119 hours or 7,140 minutes is within your control.

- You created a time-log journal to produce behavior awareness.

  These are your tools. Don't waste any more minutes lamenting your present situation. No procrastinating. Take action. It's your time, your life, and your body.

4 "I Don't Have the Energy"

A woman at a party recently asked me what I did for a living. When I told her, she started in on a tirade about how most of the other moms at her son's school dropped their kids off wearing exercise clothes. She went on and on about how these mothers seemed so happy, so capable, so thin. This obviously was an issue for her. I asked her what bugged her so much about these women. She said, "They just seem to have so much energy and I can barely get out of bed."

"Okay," I said. "Can I ask you a few questions?" She nodded. I first asked her, "Do you exercise?" She said no. I then asked, "How many hours do you sleep each night?" She said, "Oh, not enough." I asked her if she drinks water. "No," she said, "I hate it." I then asked her, "Are you interested in working with my firm in Chicago to really improve your energy level, lose weight, and feel great?" She said, "I don't know. Maybe I'll give it a try. Do you really think it could work for me?"

Three months later she was one of those moms wearing exercise clothes when she dropped her kids off at school and she had lost more than sixteen pounds.

When I conceptualized *Flip the Switch*, I constantly toyed with whether Chapter 3, "'I Don't Have the Time,'" or Chapter 4, "'I Don't Have the Energy,'" should come first. The fact is you can't increase your energy level if you don't take the time, but you need the increased energy to make the most of your time. So, which comes first? I eventually decided to help you tackle time management first so that you could find the time to exercise and learn how to take control of your food choices, and then explore the energy factor. But please do keep this in mind: Increased energy will provide you with more time. If you take or create a

> **"I DON'T FEEL GOOD."**
>
> —LUTHER BURBANK, LAST WORDS BEFORE HE DIED

small amount of additional time for yourself, you will find the benefits of doing so will include an additional burst of energy.

Trust me. As you become more fit, healthy, and lean as a result of the planning you have done to incorporate exercise and healthier, low-calorie eating into your life, you will experience the added benefit of an increase in energy. So, as you read this chapter, realize that the previous chapter on time management works in tandem with this chapter on energy. If you take nothing more from this book than the fact that energy and time work concurrently, I will feel that I have made a contribution to your ultimate decision to flip the switch.

THE MORE FIT YOU ARE, THE MORE ENERGIZED YOU WILL BE

What Is Energy?

What exactly is energy, and how can we best use it to our advantage to flip? Energy, like time, is a limited commodity that we all possess in varying degrees. Several factors play a role in depleting your energy supply, and it's important that you know how these factors work and which apply to you.

Energy-Depleting Factor #1: Excess Body Weight

Our bodies are constructed to carry a certain amount of weight. All of our bodily components—heart, lungs, muscles, bones, joints, and so on—function optimally within a lean body. Now I don't want to give you the impression that this means you have to be at a so-called perfect weight. It simply means that you should strive to keep your body as lean as possible to better assist it to function effectively. What happens when weight is added to your body? All of the body's internal organs are then required to perform their various functions for a larger amount of mass. Consequently, they must work not only harder but overtime, which expends a greater amount of energy.

EXTRA WEIGHT DRAINS ENERGY

Just so there is no confusion on this issue, the more weight you add to your body, the more energy you will have to expend to maintain that body. When you expend more energy, you are drawing upon and can deplete your body's supply of energy. Additional body weight means that life's basic activities demand more energy to perform.

Cleaning the house requires more energy, walking the dog requires more energy, playing with the kids requires more energy, shopping requires more energy, practically every physical activity you perform requires more energy. That is why, right now, if you are overweight and out of shape, you feel you have little or no energy. In fact, most of the time, you feel nearly exhausted. Am I correct?

To demonstrate this, go outside or get on a treadmill and walk briskly for about a quarter of a mile or approximately ten minutes. Immediately after you finish, take your heart rate. You do this by placing two fingers on your wrist and feeling your pulse. Then, looking at your watch, start with zero and count the beats for fifteen seconds. Remember that number. Repeat the walk, and this time hold, just hold, two five-pound weights, or an equivalent weight, in each hand. Don't swing the weights. With only ten extra pounds, feel the difference. At the conclusion of the second walk (same amount of time but holding weights), once again take your heart rate. Looking at your watch, start with zero and count the beats for fifteen seconds. Compare the heart rate produced by each walk. Which was higher? Obviously the second number was higher than the first. What this clearly demonstrates is that your heart muscle had to work considerably harder to carry the added weight. The next depleting factor in our review, decreased cardiovascularity, explores the heart muscle in detail, but for now, consider the impact added weight has on your body. Contemplate what it is like for your body with fifteen, twenty, twenty-five, thirty, thirty-five, forty, or more additional pounds. And don't forget, your body has to carry all that extra weight around all day, not just for a few minutes. And your heart has to keep supplying oxygen as you move about.

Didn't it feel great to put the two five-pound weights down? You instantly felt lighter. If you are presently overweight, imagine the exhilarating feeling and the additional energy you will possess by not being burdened by this extra weight. Once again, visualize. Close your eyes and see yourself running for the bus and not being out of breath when you get on board. So many of the people with whom I have worked over the years have said that this feeling alone was the motivation to live forever flipped.

What other role does excess body weight play in depleting our energy level? Clearly the risk of disease escalates as the body's weight increases, and with disease, our energy level is further sapped. Look back over the statistics I cited in Chapter 1. In the past decade, the number of overweight individuals in the United States has grown to more than 64.5 percent of the total American population. Concurrently, statistics point to an increase in the number of Americans afflicted by heart disease, cancer, and type II diabetes, which alone has increased more than 49 percent over the past ten years.

Don't overlook other physical damage that occurs as a result of excess weight—problems related to the back, spine, knees, and other joints of the body. Reflect on the number of your family members, friends, or colleagues who complain of back pain, who are contemplating having back surgery or even joint replacement at a relatively young age. This is not a result of simple aging. It is a direct result of carrying additional weight the human body was not designed to transport. And, yes, many times it can result from chronic overexercise, such as excessive running or step and spinning classes. More on this in Chapter 8. These diseases and injuries make continual withdrawals from our energy bank.

These factors, including an increase in the risk of disease and the resulting physical damage, force the body to compensate. By compensating, I mean that the body tries its best to adjust; it's very smart and will work harder to either fight the disease or correct the imbalance. This compensation depletes the body's energy. By eliminating

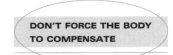

DON'T FORCE THE BODY TO COMPENSATE

the weight you eliminate a major negative force affecting your energy level. As the scale goes down, your energy level goes up—and your mental attitude will soar as the physical pain diminishes and you begin to like the way you look and feel and appreciate what you can now accomplish.

Energy-Depleting Factor 2: Decreased Cardiovascularity—Being "Out of Shape"

"Decreased cardiovascularity" is just a formal or polite euphemism for being out of shape. Saving heartbeats is one of the key components to improving your energy level. Consider the following. Walk up a flight of stairs with a group of friends. Observe those who bound up the stairs and exhibit no outward signs of fatigue or distress versus those who are panting and clearly struggling to reach the top. The former group, the fit group, is in better cardiovascular shape than the latter. The fit group bounding up the stairs also used fewer heartbeats. The unfit group, whose hearts beat more rapidly, depleted a greater amount of their energy than the fit group. You probably noticed that it takes the unfit group a few minutes to catch their breath. They are unable to move on. After just one flight of stairs they require several minutes to bring their bodies' cardiovascular system back into equilibrium.

Bank Your Energy

How do heartbeats use our energy? Energy is consumed because you have asked your heart muscle, the most important muscle of the body, to work harder. Those extra beats could have been saved for other activities or simply added to your body's "energy bank." That's right, you can actually bank your energy by not using it. This is similar to a savings account. You can spend the money you put in it or you can save it. By saving it, you will be making it available for future needs. Saving heartbeats can translate into a longer life. Once you spend the beats, like the money, they will be gone. Also, remember that money you save can be used to invest and grow. The same applies to your life. Invest in the flip and achieve significant returns on both the quality and the quantity of your life.

Why to Make the Heart Beat Faster

When the heart beats, it supplies blood throughout the body. Blood transports oxygen throughout the body. We know the human body requires an adequate supply of oxygen to function properly. Obviously, the heart works twenty-four hours a day, seven days a week pumping blood, supplying that oxygen. From the moment of conception, a fetus requires oxygen to develop; within five to six weeks, the heart muscle begins to develop and beat.

Normally, we don't want to drastically increase our heart rate, with one significant exception—during exercise. When we are out of shape, the heart has to work harder. Think back to the example about climbing the flight of stairs; you would never want to ask your heart to beat faster *except* during exercise. Cardiovascular exercise is the key to improved cardiovascularity, which means the body is transporting oxygen more efficiently. Here's how it works. Going back to my staircase example, the large muscles of the lower body, specifically the quadriceps (front of the legs), the hamstrings (back of the legs), and the gluteus maximus (your behind) need to work to propel you up each step.

These large muscles require oxygen to perform the activity. Remember, oxygen is in the blood and blood is pumped by the heart. So, as you go from step one to step two and on and on, the muscles keep demanding more oxygen-rich blood. If you perform this activity for fifteen to twenty minutes, you actually will be training your body, and specifically your heart, to respond to the activity. In other

A FIT BODY TRANSPORTS O₂ EFFICIENTLY

words, your body becomes more conditioned. Walking up these stairs for fifteen to twenty minutes is an example of cardiovascular exercise, as is walking, running, cycling, swimming, an aerobics class—in other words, any physical motion that requires the heart rate to accelerate (which additionally includes strength and resistance exercises).

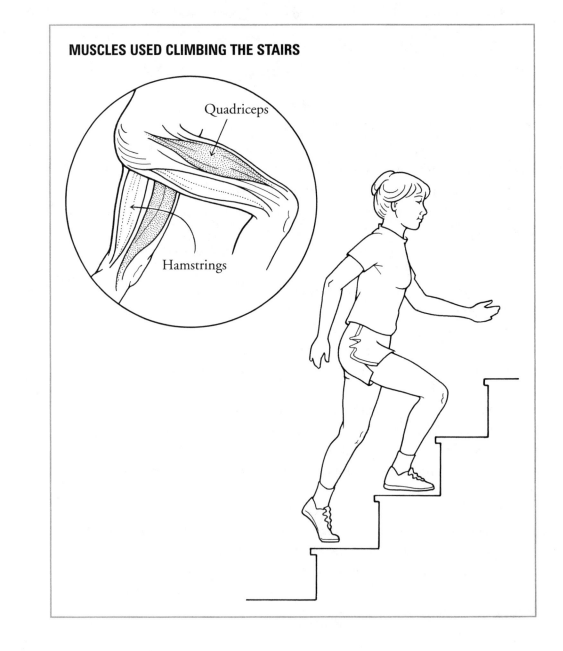

MUSCLES USED CLIMBING THE STAIRS

Quadriceps

Hamstrings

COMPONENTS OF CARDIOVASCULAR ACTIVITY

- Muscles require oxygen to perform physical activity.

- Oxygen is transported by the blood.

- Blood is pumped by the heart.

- When you perform cardiovascular activities, muscles demand more oxygen-rich blood. The heart pumps to provide that blood.

- The more efficient your cardiovascular system, the less the heart has to beat.

If you regularly perform a cardiovascular activity two to three times a week for fifteen to twenty minutes, this will greatly enhance your cardiovascularity.

I do want your heart to beat faster during cardiovascular exercise, because that will ultimately lead your heart to beat less when it is at rest. Yes, faster equals slower. Why? Your heart muscle is becoming "conditioned" to the demands you are placing upon it. This occurs because the heart becomes more efficient at supplying oxygen to the working muscles. Something called "stroke volume" improves, which means more oxygen-rich blood is pumped with each beat. Basically, you are getting "more bang for your buck" with each heartbeat.

Before I got into shape in my early twenties I was totally "deconditioned." I remember going up the flight of stairs in my fraternity house and gasping for breath at the top. I could actually be heard wheezing throughout the house. My fraternity brothers knew I was home. It always took me a few minutes to recover. And for the record, I was climbing fewer than thirty steps.

Take Your Pulse

Take your resting pulse to see whether you have improved your cardiovascular system. A resting pulse identifies the amount of beats your heart must perform to provide oxygen throughout the body when you are inactive. Ideally your resting pulse should be taken first thing in the morning while you are still lying in bed. And I must add, this is when you wake up without the alarm clock. Just the sound of an alarm can jolt your heart rate and provide an inaccurate reading.

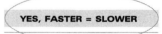
YES, FASTER = SLOWER

Do this on a weekend or a day when you don't need an alarm to awaken.

Establish Your Resting Heart Rate

Take your pulse once again as I asked you to do earlier in this chapter. You do this by placing two fingers at your wrist. Feel the beats of your heart. If you can't find it there, then try at your neck. If you can't find it there, you might consider calling 911!

Identify and record this number as you begin to change the negative factors that affect your energy level; you will see this number dramatically decline. Why? Once again, your body will need to use fewer heartbeats to supply oxygen-rich blood to the working muscles. Elite athletes are known to have resting heart rates in the forties to low fifties. Mine is around the low fifties, which is great by me, especially since my father and three of my grandparents died of heart-related complications.

A Heart "Tune-up"

Simply put, improve your heart's cardiovascular effectiveness as a supplier of oxygen throughout your body and you will conserve heartbeats and subsequently increase your energy level. Think of it as a tune-up for your heart. When you get a tune-up for your car, your car operates more efficiently and it uses fuel more efficiently. The same applies to your body. You can go the distance with less fuel. Give your heart a regular tune-up and you will experience an overwhelming difference in your energy level.

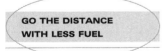

GO THE DISTANCE
WITH LESS FUEL

This can be accomplished at any age. A recent case study conducted by doctors at the University of Texas Southwestern and Presbyterian Hospital in Dallas demonstrated that in just six months of regular aerobic exercise, fifty-year-olds were able to achieve the fitness levels they had at the age of twenty. Just know, it's never too late.

Energy-Depleting Factor 3: Diminished Physical Strength

After the age of twenty, the average person loses between one-half to seven-tenths of a pound of muscle each year. That equals five to seven pounds of muscle loss each decade. Why is this significant? Because diminished muscle equates to diminished physical strength. And when you lack physical strength you lack energy. If your physical strength is diminished, everything becomes harder: carrying groceries from the car, holding your child, taking the garbage out, and the countless other daily tasks that require physical strength. I can recall in my out-of-shape teens and early twenties when activities such as carrying luggage through an airport, packing the trunk of my car, shoveling snow, or moving a small piece of furniture tired me out. Simple daily activities rapidly depleted my energy bank. I was spending, spending, spending. Now that I have rebuilt my strength, the majority of these tasks are effortless. In fact, I rarely think about them.

Recall my earlier statement that less muscle equals less strength, but aging has relatively little to do with decreased strength. An individual's behavior is the principal factor—and the behavior I'm referring to is inactivity. *Muscle loss and the resulting energy level depletion that occurs are not inevitable.* Correct strength and resistance training dramatically halts this deterioration process (see Chapter 8). If you have read my previous book, *The Business Plan for the Body,* skimmed one of my newspaper or magazine articles, or seen me on television, you know that I am fully committed to strength training as the key to weight loss and vastly improved energy levels. Also, note that getting strong has a powerful effect on both your body and your mind.

According to Jack Raglin, associate professor of kinesiology at Indiana University, "Exercise produces a cocktail of chemicals and a whole host of physical and psychological changes." Bottom line, if

LACK OF PHYSICAL STRENGTH = LACK OF ENERGY

BEHAVIOR, NOT AGE, AFFECTS STRENGTH

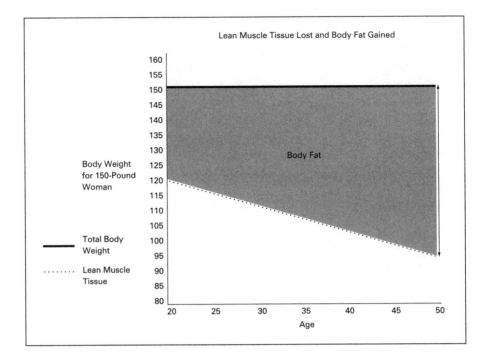

Lean Muscle Tissue Lost and Body Fat Gained

Body Fat

Body Weight for 150-Pound Woman

——— Total Body Weight

.... Lean Muscle Tissue

Age

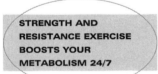

STRENGTH AND
RESISTANCE EXERCISE
BOOSTS YOUR
METABOLISM 24/7

you feel better, you will possess more energy. Once again here is an instance where the mind and the body work in tandem to produce the most dramatic results.

In Chapter 8, "'I Hate to Exercise,'" I will describe in detail the many benefits of strength and resistance exercise, as well as provide specific workouts that you can do. For now, just remember that strength and resistance exercise is the *only* form of exercise that boosts your metabolism twenty-four hours a day, seven days a week. This will dramatically assist you in weight loss and in dealing with the first energy-depleting factor I addressed, excess body weight. So, realize that strength and resistance exercise is not only about wearing a size 8 or acquiring six-pack abdominals, it's also about dramatically increasing your energy level.

Energy-Depleting Factor 4: Sleep Deprivation

Sleep is an essential ingredient in enhancing your energy level. The only time the body has a chance to repair, rejuvenate, and process is during sleep. Without adequate rest, the body cannot function effectively. This is especially pertinent given the fact that sleep deprivation is on the rise in the United States. *Consumer Reports on Health* states that "sleeping just half an hour less than you need can make you feel less alert the next day; sleeping an hour less can impair mental and physical performance as much as two alcoholic drinks can." Some evidence suggests that inadequate sleep may weaken the body's immune system. Other recent research suggests that even moderate, chronic sleep debt may increase the risk of developing insulin resistance, a condition that predisposes people to diabetes, as well as high blood pressure, coronary heart disease, stroke, and possibly cancer. Lack of sleep may also inhibit nocturnal surges of growth hormone, and in theory, contribute to weight gain and reductions in muscle mass.

Finally, sleep deprivation reduces the production of leptin. Leptin, the subject of numerous case studies, is a hormone that signals the body to stop fueling, or eating, when it is full. Research shows that certain obese individuals have low leptin levels and certain lean individuals have high leptin levels. Therefore, researchers now realize that there is a correlation between leptin and body weight. At present, those researchers are in the process of determining how optimal leptin levels can be achieved. Thus, we know that sleep deprivation can reduce leptin production, which can be harmful to your health, your weight, and your energy level.

In addition, many clients have told me that they eat when they are tired during the day to boost their energy level. Sound familiar? Eating candy during the day to get a sugar boost, sipping on lattes or cappuccinos to give you both a caffeine and a sugar boost, popping in cookies at the office or in the car to keep you alert. I have heard all of this (and more) over the years from people who are trying to stay awake and alert throughout the day. Avoid these cravings by starting the day rested. Try it. You will be amazed by the results a good night's sleep can produce. Sleep experts say that seven to eight hours gets the job done.

Find the Time to Sleep

Sleep deprivation is lessened with proper time management. Go back over your time-log journal in Chapter 3 and determine where you can

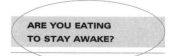

CHRONIC SLEEP DEPRIVATION MAY INCREASE YOUR RISK OF DISEASE

"I DON'T HAVE THE ENERGY"

79

ARE YOU EATING TO STAY AWAKE?

For years clients have been telling me that their worst eating behavior occurs late at night. Many of the very successful, hard-working individuals I know eat half of their calories before 10:00 P.M. and half of them after 10:00 P.M. They eat perfectly during the day, starting off with fruit and yogurt, a small salad with some grilled chicken at lunch, poached salmon with steamed broccoli at dinner—and then a pint of Häagen-Dazs and a bag of cookies during Letterman. Why? Many times, it is a conditioned response or simply the only time they have to themselves all day. As they relax and unwind in front of the television or with a book, the "comfort" eating occurs. To avoid this, try to get into bed earlier, *without* food; you will find that you are saving yourself hundreds of calories each day and start to see the weight come off. Or, if you do like to snack before bed, try a lower-calorie option, such as baby carrots, air-popped popcorn, a piece of fruit, or a ½ cup of low-fat frozen yogurt.

make some adjustments that would enable you to go to bed earlier. Remember, I said that this book was designed to incorporate some of the elements of a workbook. You can keep all your information in one place and you can review and adjust it accordingly. One small note with regard to getting to bed earlier: You do not have to do this at the expense of others. If you manage your time wisely, you can take care of your family, spouse, or parent *and* yourself simultaneously.

Energy-Depleting Factor 5: Dehydration

A human being's body is composed of nearly 70 percent water. Water, after oxygen, is the body's single most important element. It performs a role in most bodily functions: It regulates the body's temperature, removes waste, transports nutrients, including oxygen, to our cells, cushions our joints, and protects organs and tissues. Being severely dehydrated can dangerously affect kidney function, our circulatory system, and digestion. Properly hydrated, the body functions optimally. When the body is dehydrated, it is out of balance. Once again, when your body is out of balance, it needs to expend more energy to attempt to rebalance.

H₂O IS THE BODY'S
SECOND MOST
IMPORTANT ELEMENT

Interested in Metabolizing Fat?

In addition, your body needs water in order to efficiently metabolize stored fat. When you shortchange your water supply, you're likely to slow down that process, meaning it's more difficult for you to turn stored body fat into energy, or calories. Why take the time and energy to lose weight, only to slow the process down by not properly hydrating your body? It just doesn't make sense. Drink!

Sodium and Water Balance

Why *are* so many Americans dehydrated? There are two reasons. First, sodium. We eat out more than ever. Restaurant food is loaded with sodium. I have watched chefs in open kitchens use huge salt shakers to salt everything. Did you know that many salads in restaurants are salted before the dressing is placed on top? Listed below are a few popular products that contain a high amount of sodium per serving. Keep in mind, Americans have been advised by experts to consume no more than 2,500 milligrams of sodium each day.

8 ounces of V8 Juice	800 milligrams
8 ounces of canned chicken noodle soup	910 milligrams
1 tablespoon of soy sauce	892 milligrams
½ cup of canned green beans (½ cup of frozen green beans contains 0 milligrams)	360 milligrams
One-quarter of a 12-inch frozen pepperoni pizza	1,000 milligrams
½ cup of low-fat cottage cheese	470 milligrams
1 McDonald's Regular Cheeseburger	830 milligrams

Read Labels for Sodium Content

If you take a moment to read labels on some of your favorite products, you may be shocked to see the high levels of sodium. For example, almost all soups are enormously high in sodium with the exception of low-sodium varieties or soups that you make at home.

Feel the Bloat

When you consume excess sodium, your body will retain a good deal of water to dilute the sodium concentration. And studies confirm that the more salt people consume, the more fluid will be excreted by the kidneys. This in turn causes the body to become further dehydrated and consequently "out of balance" as the water is both fighting to deal with all the excess sodium and being excreted by the kidneys. Water is not being used to hydrate the rest of the body and assist it to function optimally. The only way to reverse this trend is to limit your sodium intake and drink more water. I can't tell you how many people say to me, "Oh, I can't drink water because I am already bloated. Drinking more will only make it worse." That is totally wrong. By drinking water, you will eliminate the bloat. Your body will say, "Okay, there is water available. Release the reserves." You start to eliminate the stored water and the puffiness disappears. Drinking water (and eating foods with a high water content, such as fruits and vegetables) is the only way to keep the body in balance.

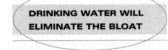

DRINKING WATER WILL
ELIMINATE THE BLOAT

Americans and H₂O Rarely Meet

Americans simply do not drink very much water. I observe people at lunches, dinners, parties, even while working out, and I rarely see them drinking water. I see them drinking soda, coffee, alcohol, sports drinks, and juice, but rarely water. Why is this so important? Because, as previously noted, the human body is predominantly composed of water. If you stop reading right now and pour yourself a large glass of water, you will immediately begin to increase your energy level as your body will operate more efficiently when properly hydrated. Your body will no longer have to struggle as hard to maintain water balance. Now repeat that eight, ten, twelve times a day and you will really begin to feel the difference.

Is Eight Enough or Too Much?

I'm well aware of the controversy, reported in the media, regarding the standard rule of drinking eight eight-ounce glasses of water each day, for a total of sixty-four ounces of water. What the media fails to report is that you have to consider your size, your activity level, your sodium intake (most Americans consume twice the recommended amount), the climate you live in, and the medications you may be taking when determining how much water your body requires on a daily basis. All of these affect your water balance. If you live in a dry climate (the dryness depletes your water balance), drink alcohol (as alcohol breaks down in the body, water is used in the process), exercise regularly (the body cools off by perspiration, which throws off water), or take certain medications, then you should be drinking *more* water because all of these factors deplete your water balance. You definitely should be drinking more water if you are larger (taller or heavier) because you have more body mass to hydrate.

Don't Play Water Games

FREQUENT HEADACHES CAN INDICATE DEHYDRATION

I want to make a quick point about water balance and weight loss. Most crash, gimmicky diets immediately play with your body's water balance. That is why the scale goes down so quickly. Did you lose five pounds in five days? No. You probably lost one pound of fat and four pounds of water. The minute you go off of the diet, you will gain those four pounds back. Clients and friends constantly ask me why the scale is jumping around so much. Ninety-nine times out of a hundred, they are not consistently drinking approximately the same amount of water.

So, establish an amount of water each day that feels right for you. For some, it may be forty or fifty ounces. For others—myself included, given that I am very active, six feet tall, frequently fly (check out the next section, below), and drink wine on occasion—it will be about one hundred ounces.

"I DON'T HAVE THE ENERGY"

83

WATER PILLS

A water pill (a diuretic) is one of the worst things you can take when you are bloated. Here is the scenario: You are bloated because you probably consumed too little water or too much sodium, or if you're a woman, this may happen just before your period. You are holding on to too much water because you are dehydrated. So, by taking a water pill, you force water out of your body. Guess what? You just made matters worse as the body will now bloat even *more*. Avoid taking these pills. Only a diuretic pill prescribed by a medical professional (often to combat high blood pressure) should be taken.

SWEAT IS GOOD

I just touched upon the point of perspiration during exercise. People frequently tell me that they don't sweat. A very attractive sixty-year-old woman, who had been raised in Atlanta, said to me at her initial consultation in a wonderful southern accent, "I simply don't sweat." I observed that she didn't drink any water. Then, once I had her drinking more water, she was shocked. She couldn't understand why she was sweating. I explained to her that her body was so dehydrated before that she didn't have any water to throw off. Now, properly hydrated, her body was doing what it was meant to do when it overheated—sweat. For the record, she also complained of chronic headaches (frequently a result of dehydration) and mentioned to me one day that they had subsided. I pointed out that now she was properly hydrated. Water makes such a difference.

Other Dehydrating Factors

There are several other factors that contribute to dehydration. Research has shown that airline cabin pressure can deplete an individual's water balance by as much as 32 ounces an hour. For a two-hour flight, that would equate to 64 ounces; for a cross-country flight, more than 120 ounces. Think of what can occur when you travel overseas. Many of you may have experienced the headache, nausea, or fatigue that result from flying but were not aware of the cause. The chances are great that the cause was dehydration. Please, drink as much water as possible on a plane. You might consider buying some and carrying it on since I have noticed that many airlines have cut back on the amount of water served on flights. Notice they are never out of soda!

One out of ten elderly individuals (those seventy and older) are hospitalized because they are dehydrated. This occurs because, as individuals age, the effectiveness of the thirst mechanism in the body diminishes. Consequently, they don't feel thirsty and drink less fluids. If you, a friend, or a family member is getting older, be aware of this phenomenon and encourage proper hydration. Don't wait for thirst to be your guide. The thirst mechanism kicks in when you are already thirty-two ounces down in water. Therefore, you have to drink four eight-ounce glasses of water to just get your body back into balance. Don't wait for thirst to be your guide, just keep drinking.

Can Other Beverages Count Toward Hydration?

This is a subject of continual debate. Beverages that contain caffeine, such as coffee, tea, or soda, provide a small amount of water; how-

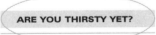

ever, they also act as a diuretic. Diuretics flush water out of the body, which is exactly what you do *not* want. Therefore, if you do drink beverages other than water, be aware of this effect. Also note that if you are drinking juice, sports drinks, or nondiet soda, you are consuming many calories (much more on this in Chapter 7). You should consider diluting these beverages with water or just reaching for water in the first place.

A further guide to hydration is the color of your urine. Clear urine is an indication that you are properly hydrated. If your urine is dark or yellow, then most likely you are dehydrated. (This is the general rule; however, taking certain medications may alter the color of your urine.)

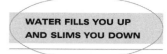

WATCH THE CALORIES IN SODA, JUICE, AND SPORTS DRINKS

Hungry or Thirsty?

I find that people often misinterpret thirst for hunger. Instead of grabbing a glass or bottle of water, many will grab something to eat. Think about that for a moment. Being persistently dehydrated can cause you to eat excessively (see energy-depleting factor number six). The next time you find yourself at the refrigerator, a snack cart, or a convenience/grocery store, stop and ask yourself, "Am I hungry or am I thirsty?" You might find that water could totally satisfy this craving. And by the way, water also helps to fill you up, so you will feel less hungry.

"I DON'T HAVE THE ENERGY"

85

Food and Water

Does food ever count as water? Yes. High-water-content foods, such as fruits and vegetables, definitely contribute to your water balance. The more you consume fruits and vegetables, the more you add nutrients and vitamins to your body *and* enhance your water balance. As you will see, fruits and vegetables should be the foundation of your weight-loss eating plan.

WATER FILLS YOU UP AND SLIMS YOU DOWN

Energy-Depleting Factor 6: Excessive Eating

Ten to 15 percent of our daily caloric burning is the direct result of the digestive process. When you eat excessively, you are asking your stomach to constantly keep digesting food. This severely affects your energy level. Try the following as an experiment. Go to Chapter 7, "'I Love to Eat,'" and follow the *Flip the Switch* Seven-Day Jump-Start Eating Plan. Eat those foods for one week, drink sixty-four ounces of water daily, and carefully monitor how you feel. You will feel a significant increase in your energy level because you will not be devoting as much energy to digestion. Plus, your body will be functioning in a properly hydrated environment. Trust me, this makes a significant difference in both your energy level and how you feel.

CONSTANT EATING
MAKES YOU TIRED

Careful Combining

In addition to curbing excessive eating, exercise caution when it comes to combining too many different foods. (I am not referring to the unsupported theory that you should not combine protein and carbohydrate in the same meal. That theory is totally false, with no medical evidence to support it. If you would like a detailed analysis of fad diets, then take a look at Chapter 2 of *The Business Plan for the Body*, "The Competition.") The fact is that simple food choices will boost your energy level. To test this, have some grilled chicken with steamed broccoli and a medium-size baked potato; on another occasion go to a buffet table and sample many different dishes. Even if the buffet's calorie count is equal to that of the grilled chicken, broccoli, and potato, you will feel a diminishment in your energy level after consuming too broad a variety of foods. This is because so much of your body's energy is being used to digest this "banquet." Keep it simple; save some of that energy you've been currently using for digestion.

If you still can't relate to this idea, consider how you feel after a big holiday feast. Do you feel energized? You know and I know that the answer is a resounding no.

Energy-Depleting Factor Number 7: Lack of Sun

Circadian rhythm is the body's natural pattern of waking and sleeping that occurs within a twenty-four-hour day. Regular exposure to the sun can help maintain a normal sleep-wake cycle. Some sunshine can be helpful in lessening sleep deprivation. The sun also plays a critical role in our mood. Seasonal affective disorder, or SAD, is a disorder experienced by some people when their body's circadian rhythm, or so-called biological clock, has difficulty adjusting to the shortage of sunlight in the wintertime. Many times this leads to anxiety, an increased craving of carbohydrates, and an overall feeling of depression and unhappiness. This may result in your eating more and exercising less. Once again, you are going the wrong way. In other words, you should be exercising more and eating less. Approximately 25 percent of the population suffer some degree of SAD while 5 percent may experience a more severe form. If you feel you may be one of these people, then consult your physician; he or she may prescribe phototherapy, which simulates sunlight and can reset circadian rhythm.

Energy-Depleting Factor 8: Negative Thoughts

Now I am going to ask you to consider your energy level as a function of your mind as well as your body. We can all recall times in our lives when we were consumed by a negative situation, whether it was a bad relationship, problems at work, money issues, or a family crisis. While I am not a psychotherapist trained to deal with these issues, I can say that I have spent more than fifteen years working with clients for three to four hours each week, meeting with them one-on-one, and have observed the damaging effects of negative thoughts on their energy levels.

I have seen people who were virtually consumed by negative thoughts; they were mentally, and in some instances nearly physically, paralyzed. Their energy levels were totally sapped. All of their energy was focused on the negative aspects of their lives. They had little or no energy left for other tasks or other people. How do you find a way to maneuver yourself out of these difficult situations? Unfortunately, there is no easy answer. I can't say I know for certain or that one bit of advice applies to every situation, but I can say that negative thoughts are certainly a significant drain on one's energy level.

Be Optimistic, Feel Stronger, Live Longer

In Chapters 1 and 2, I urged you to explore both the emotional and the physical aspects of your past and present life; now take a moment

"YOU'VE GOT TO ACCENTUATE THE POSITIVE, ELIMINATE THE NEGATIVE . . ."

to think about those issues that might be depleting your energy today. Years ago, Mayo Clinic researchers found that people who were optimists in their youth tended to live twelve years longer than pessimists. So, to "get happy" (which I talk about more in Chapter 10), here is an exercise that will help you deal with those negative thoughts. See the sidebar on page 89.

A thought log is basically a journal in which you catalog anything negative that you are dealing with in your present life. Be specific and prioritize your worries and problems. Begin with the one topic that troubles you the most, then continue in descending order of importance through each and every issue. The following categories, not necessarily in this order, tend to be the ones that most individuals dwell upon:

1. Family safety

2. Work/professional issues

3. Why me?

4. Appearance

5. Lack of love/respect

6. Self-esteem

7. Economics/financial security

We all have some of these problems—that's a normal part of life. The question is, do these concerns enter our minds so frequently that they deplete our energy? Normal worries are one thing, but if those cares escalate into obsessive negative thoughts, they can become quite destructive. Mental health professionals have long noted the mind's ability to ignore reality, especially where one's self is concerned. You may be unaware of the impact that negative thoughts are having on you. But you should be aware that bad situations and negative thoughts *do* deplete a considerable amount of your energy. Just knowing that there is a relationship between energy and negative thinking

IF YOU GAIN INSIGHT,
YOU'LL GAIN CONTROL

will help you considerably, and that's the reason for your thought log.

Is This Stuff Worth Worrying About?

Examine what you have written in the space at right. How big are your worries? How insurmountable are your problems? All of your concerns are probably "realistic"—the question is, are they worth worrying over? It's easy to dismiss or put into perspective the small stuff, but what about the really big stuff? Weigh the pros and cons and the reality of each worry. Use your thought log as you used your time-log journal. Gain insight. See the reality in black and white and start dealing with the issues rather than avoiding them. You and I both know that if you don't deal with issues, they won't go away. They simply live inside of us and usually get worse, until *we* decide to take control.

And if you have a truly damaging problem such as a job loss, a family member with a terminal illness, or a substance-abuse problem that requires professional intervention, then by all means get help.

Energy-Depleting Factor 9: Stress

A special issue of *Newsweek* magazine in 2001 reported that "stress wreaks havoc on organs from the heart to the brain." Research indicates that when you are faced with a stressful situation or activity, in addition to the known mental negative effects of stress, a physiological phenomenon occurs: Your adrenal glands release a hormone called cortisol. High cortisol levels have been linked to triggering food cravings. Overweight individuals, especially those who

"I DON'T HAVE THE ENERGY"

Create a Thought Log

carry the majority of their body fat in their midsections, as well as normal-weight individuals who seem to carry a "spare tire" around their midsections, appear to have elevated levels of cortisol in their bloodstreams.

Once Again, Explore Your Past

Studies show that high levels of stress often occur in individuals who had traumatic childhood experiences. Are your past experiences affecting your present stress levels? High cortisol levels and excess body weight go hand in hand. Come to terms with the past, eliminate the stress, lower your cortisol levels, and watch your weight drop. You will also minimize the risk of certain diseases associated with high levels of cortisol, such as cardiovascular disease, high blood pressure, diabetes, and even depression. If you have any concerns about cortisol, then consult your physician. Just know that the problem is not cortisol itself, but the manner in which you are dealing with stress.

IS FOOD A FRIEND?

Keep exploring your emotional relationship to food. How often do you think about food? Identify behaviors such as eating candy during a stressful afternoon with the kids, or breaking out the cookies when you get home from a tough day at work, or climbing into bed feeling lonely with both Ben *and* Jerry. If you can start to identify the emotional factors surrounding overeating, you will greatly increase your ability to flip.

CRAVING BROCCOLI?

According to Adam Drewnowski, Ph.D., "Food cravings arise to satisfy emotional needs, such as calming stress and reducing anxiety. The foods that gratify that emotional component typically contain fat, sugar or both. The fat or sugar in foods like chocolate, potato chips, ice cream and cookies make them taste good, explaining why we get excited about them— and why we don't typically crave skim milk, spinach or broccoli without cheese sauce." If you reduce stress, then you reduce the likelihood that you will crave and overeat high-calorie foods.

PUTTING IT ALL TOGETHER TO FLIP

A successful flip requires energy. Many factors can deplete our energy supply, including the following:

- Excess body weight
- Decreased cardiovascularity
- Diminished physical strength
- Sleep deprivation
- Dehydration
- Excessive eating
- Lack of sun
- Negative thoughts
- Stress

You can successfully manage all of these factors by thoughtful planning. If you energize your mind, then your physical energy will dramatically increase as well. Begin by creating a thought log.

5 "I Don't Have the Money"

There is one question I get about a dozen times a week. Someone will produce a bottle of pills from his or her purse, briefcase, or gym bag and ask the following question: "What do you think of these?" What the person is holding are not prescription medications but over-the-counter pills with names such as "fat burners" or "metabolism enhancers." The cost of these so-called magic pills is astounding: $20, $30, $40 or more a bottle. My response is invariably the same: "Did you really think that these would work?" Each time the answer is the same: "No, not really, but I was desperate. The people in the ad I saw just look so fit. These pills must do something."

I always urge these individuals to return the "magic" pills, get their money back, and spend some of it on exercise equipment. I recommend that they buy some strength and resistance exercise tubing, or free weights, or even a one-month membership to a health club or gym. Spend your money on products or services that work instead of ones that only give you false hope and reward you with disappointment when they don't work.

To Have or Not to Have
To Spend or Not to Spend

Whenever I hear the excuse "I don't have the money," my response is, "Do you really not *have* the money, or do you simply not want to *spend* the money?"

Let's tackle the second part of my question first, because that is frequently the real issue; we'll revisit the first part later in this chapter. Ask yourself, "Is it simply that I don't want to *spend* the money?" I am going to make an assumption. I'm sure you've spent money trying to lose weight in the past, and nothing happened. You didn't lose the weight. You couldn't fit into that outfit you bought a size smaller in anticipation of losing weight. You didn't feel better. You didn't look better. No one noticed any change; you felt defeated, and you felt as if you'd wasted your money. You gave up. Sound familiar? It probably does. All of us, myself included (remember my Wonder Weighted Belt?), have spent money on some crazy pill, program, or machine that was supposed to be the answer to weight loss. They didn't work. None of them. We felt taken advantage of and foolish, and vowed never to spend money on weight loss again. We've all become skeptical and cynical in part because of all the hype—"Lose 10 Pounds this Weekend!!!"—that exists in the weight-loss marketplace.

A Gimmick Is a Gimmick

We were looking for an easy solution to weight loss. But all the quick-fix pills, devices, and potions are doomed to fail because they are based on gimmicks that don't work. Just channel-surf in the middle of the night—it seems as if virtually every other infomercial has something to do with weight loss. These infomercials promote "metabolism"-boosting pills and exercise machines that make one ridiculous exaggerated claim after another. I am always researching these products for my books, business, and lectures and can honestly tell you that they rarely work. While I am saving my analysis of metabolism for the next chapter, I will say that most pills don't raise your metabolism and the few that do can cause significant damage to your body, especially your heart muscle. Remember Fen-Phen? If you had carefully read or listened to the advertisements for these weight-loss products, you would have seen that all the results they cited were achieved by individuals who took the pill or used the product *and followed a low-calorie eating and exercise program.* This information is usually buried in the small print on the bottom of the advertisement or quickly flashed across the television screen.

Could you have achieved similar results by following a low-calorie eating and exercise program? Absolutely. The pill and the equipment were unnecessary. Don't be embarrassed. We have all fallen prey to the

LOSING WEIGHT
SHOULDN'T BE EXPENSIVE

seductive power of advertising. Just don't let that happen this time with your desire and belief that you can lose weight. To succeed at weight loss, you have to be realistic and disciplined. Go back to exercise 5 in Chapter 1: "I believed in my ability to be successful in achieving my goal of . . ." You were most likely realistic and disciplined in that endeavor. Now apply those same tools and techniques to weight loss. Yes, overcoming weight issues is a complicated task, but it's not an impossible, expensive task.

It Didn't Look so Hard on TV

Most exercise machines and gadgets purchased through infomercials are considerably more difficult to operate at home than they appear to be in the commercial. Once the machine arrives, you can't figure it out. It doesn't look the same way it did on the infomercial; it looks flimsy. Many are nearly impossible to assemble and use. I have been in the fitness industry for more than sixteen years and have been presented with equipment that I have absolutely no idea how to assemble and operate. The instructions are vague, confusing, and many times incomplete. Consequently, the machine sits there, collecting dust, providing service as a clothes rack, taking up room—a constant reminder that you wasted your money. You feel duped. It's depressing. These products are always presented as inexpensive. Rarely is the total price highlighted; rather, you see $39.95 in three easy payments plus shipping and handling. This ends up costing you more than $140. That is a good deal of money and far more than is necessary to spend to create an effective exercise plan. In addition, much of this equipment is potentially unsafe.

In Chapter 2 we explored the power of positive visualization. But *negative visualization* can also have an impact—one that you'll want to avoid. Seeing these dud products in your home becomes a *negative visual,* a constant reminder of your failure once again at weight loss. You spent money and derived no benefit. Do yourself a big favor. Throw out that piece of exercise equipment sitting in your bedroom, basement, or garage. If it's a safe piece of machinery, donate it, get the tax deduction, and save some money. Get rid of the reminder that you spent money and failed at weight loss. I want only positive reminders and positive energy to flow through your home.

IS YOUR EXERCISE MACHINE COLLECTING A LOT OF DUST?

Are You a Member of the Club?

What about health club or gym memberships? A client's assistant and I were having a talk one day about New Year's resolutions. She said, "Do you know what my resolution is this year? My resolution is to quit paying for my health club that I never use. The next time I join a gym, I am going to commit myself to using it rather than wasting my money." Now, in the privacy of your home, raise your hand if you ever joined a health club. Now, briefly in your head, count how many times you actually went to that club. Probably not many. I know that some of the biggest heath club operations in the country admit that only about 20 percent of their members frequently visit the club. The other 80 percent just continue to pay their monthly or yearly dues and rarely if ever use the facilities. The existence of most health clubs is predicated on the fact that the majority of the membership will not use the club. If you are a part of this nonuser majority, then clearly it is a complete waste of money. On the other hand, if you do go to the club regularly, you can readily appreciate the value of the membership expenditure. Later in this chapter we'll review the ins and outs of health club memberships.

> MOST GYMS HOPE YOU NEVER SHOW UP

I'm Not Going to Be Duped Again

So you see, many times the excuse "I don't have the money" really isn't the case. What so many individuals are saying is that they *do* have the money, but they have spent the money—in fact, many times they've spent considerable sums of money on weight loss and derived no return on their investment. They felt that they were "taken" and now feel foolish. For this group, it's not so much "I don't have the money" as it is "I'm not going to get duped again." Are you one of these people?

But wait a minute, what about those of you who really *don't* have the money? I'm aware that many people live on a tight budget, have a fixed income, or already have accumulated substantial debt. If money truly is a real issue for you, complete the following exercise to determine if you can find the funds to apply toward flipping. Read on—I think most of you will be pleasantly surprised to find out what this exercise will reveal.

"I DON'T HAVE THE MONEY"

Prepare a Monthly Budget

For those of you who have never constructed a monthly budget, it's much easier than you probably think. Begin by recording your total approximate monthly *after-tax income.*

To determine your monthly income, take your weekly paycheck amount (the net, not the gross), multiply it by fifty-two, since there are fifty-two weeks in a year, and then divide by twelve, since there are twelve months in a year. This amount is your monthly after-tax, or net, income. (If you are paid every other week, multiply by twenty-six, or by the total of pay periods you have. Then divide by twelve.)

Next, total all of your fixed monthly expenses. The following are examples of typical fixed monthly expenses:

Rent or mortgage

Car payment

Other loan repayments

Gasoline expense for car

Car insurance

Basic home phone service, not including long distance

Basic cellular phone service

Internet provider/cable television

Average grocery bill

Gas and electric utilities

Educational expenses

Medical insurance (do not include if directly deducted from your paycheck)

Other insurance

Predetermined savings plan (do not include 401K or any other plan if deducted automatically from your paycheck)

Total these category amounts and any other regular fixed expenses you might have identified and subtract them from your net monthly income. The remaining amount is your net monthly income *after* fixed expenses. Now determine your monthly variable expenses. Variable expenses tend to fluctuate (you have much more control over these) and include the following:

Additional phone expenses, such as long distance

Entertainment and travel

Clothes

Leisure/recreational activities, such as a sport or a hobby

Variable credit card payments

Total your variable expenses and deduct them from your net monthly income after fixed expenses. This amount represents your net monthly disposable income *after* fixed and variable expenses.

Did You Find the Funds to Flip?

Once you obtain the total of your monthly expenses, then you can better identify funds available to spend on flipping. Or, after completing the exercise, you may realize, possibly for the first time, why you are frequently broke or in debt. You may finally see that you are spending more money than you are making. This in itself is helpful since being chronically in debt can make you anxious and depressed and contribute to some of the negative thoughts and energy depletion we discussed in Chapter 4. Remember, this frustration and depression can lead you to eat even more.

Now you can determine if you do have any disposable income to devote to the flip. As you will see, the cost of exercise basics is not exorbitant. In Chapter 7, "'I Love to Eat,'" you will learn that following a healthier, low-calorie eating plan need not require much additional expense and in many instances is less expensive. If you truly don't have any extra money to invest in some simple and inexpensive tools for flipping, then it may be necessary to reduce expenses or go to the other side of the equation and explore making more money. Please don't think that I believe this is easy. But just remember, you can decide to flip the switch for a myriad of reasons—from getting your career back on track to improving your personal relationships—not just for weight loss. If you do decide that you want to flip, no matter your objective, then it's time to learn to manage and overcome those barriers that have always kept you from flipping in the past.

How Cutting Calories Will Cut Your Food Costs

Okay, you've decided to flip to get control of your weight. You believe in your ability; you visualize yourself leaner and more attractive; you determined that, yes, you do have the time to exercise and make better food choices; and you realize that your energy level will improve. Did you know that flipping can actually save you money? Obviously, eating less will help you to save money. If you stop and count all the things you eat throughout the day, you may identify quite a bit of money spent on a doughnut here or a Danish there plus all those "designer" coffee drinks. All of these treats add up. You will also save money when it comes to the sheer quantity of food eaten. When you cut down on calories, you will see your grocery bills decreasing. You will start ordering less in restaurants and opt for an appetizer and a salad rather than a big expensive entrée. All of these points will help you to save money. In addition, when you plan what you are going to eat, as I encourage you to do in Chapter 3, you are less apt to get caught hungry in an environment where expensive food is the only option or at the supermarket with a bagful of expensive, ready-to-eat, high-calorie, high-fat foods that you had never planned to buy in the first place.

You may spend more money on some foods, such as increased amounts of fresh produce. But if you stay in season and don't purchase extravagant berries or exotic high-priced fruits, you won't notice a cost increase. And keep in mind, you are probably going to be purchasing *less* food overall.

I buy huge quantities of frozen fruits and vegetables. They are easy to buy in bulk, frequently on sale, and they rarely spoil. Case studies conclusively demonstrate that many frozen fruits and vegetables retain even more vitamins and nutrients than fresh. Don't feel you are losing any of the benefits of fruits and vegetables by opting for frozen, which can prove to be a less expensive alternative to fresh. However, try to avoid canned vegetables, even if you are lured by the prices, as they are generally loaded with sodium. If you do buy them, make sure to rinse them off before eating them to minimize the sodium content.

FRESH ISN'T THE ONLY OPTION

Investing in Exercise

Let's take a look at the costs of the workouts I will take you through in Chapter 8, as well as the economics of joining a gym. The costs of your exercise program will be determined by *how* you work out and *where* you work out.

SPRI Xertubes/Xerings or Free Weights

For the at-home exerciser, my first workout program in Chapter 8 (see page 190) utilizes SPRI brand exercise tubing, which will cost you approximately $10 a tube or ring, plus the SPRI Resist-A-Ball ($29), and a SPRI small pump ($15). The second exercise program (see page 201) is done exclusively with free weights, the Resist-A-Ball, and a SPRI pump. When purchased either over the Internet or at a store, plain free weights should be priced in the vicinity of $.50 a pound. Fancy chrome weights generally are about $2 a pound. You can always start with a few weights and add more as your program progresses, or opt for an adjustable set. You can even let your family and friends know that you would appreciate holiday or birthday gifts of exercise equipment. Remember not to be enticed by expensive products available through infomercials that promise instant results.

Should You Join a Health Club or Gym?

These days, health clubs and gyms are like cars. They range from bare-bones to ultimate luxury spas. Determine what price range you can

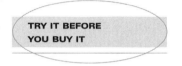
TRY IT BEFORE
YOU BUY IT

afford, then do some comparison shopping. In New York, I make it a habit to go to all of the different gyms in Manhattan so that I can observe and be aware of the latest equipment, training techniques, or trends. I have paid anywhere from $10 to $50 for a one-day membership. You'll discover a huge range in health club fees. But keep in mind, it's not the club, exercise room, or equipment that matters, it's the application—how you use your exercise time.

To help you decide whether or not to join a gym, go back to the time-log journal you completed in Chapter 3. This will enable you to determine where you decide to exercise—home or club. If you decide on a gym or club, should it be close to your home, office, or both? Once again, only you can decide.

Here's a tip: If you want to try a club, tell the club management you are in from out of town and would like to have a one-week or one-month membership. They rarely will turn you down. This enables you to check out the equipment, the members, the cleanliness, the availability of the equipment, peak versus off-peak usage, available instruction, and so on. You can decide if this is the best place for you without having to sign a long-term agreement. And if you do decide to join, take the time to fully read the contract and make it a point to identify the cancellation clause, the late-payment fees, guest fees, and finance charges, since they can be tricky. By thinking and planning you will definitely save yourself money.

Penny Wise, Pound Foolish

Whether you don't *want* to spend the money or don't *have* the money to spend, one fact is certain: If you don't invest the time, energy, and money required to flip, you may subject yourself and your loved ones to a very high future financial cost. Being overweight and out of shape can carry a huge price tag: an increase in health care and prescription drug costs; a decrease in employment productivity; an early death, leaving spouse and children behind; missed work; and missed opportunities. Realize that the investment you make today to flip will save you hundreds, if not thousands, of dollars in the years to come. We all look for profits from our investments. Rarely is any investment guaranteed, but this one is.

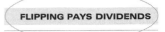

FLIPPING PAYS DIVIDENDS

PUTTING IT ALL TOGETHER TO FLIP

- Determine whether you really don't *have* the money to spend on flipping, or simply do not want to *spend* the money.

- Avoid the negative visualization that results from previous exercise purchases.

- Prepare a monthly budget to gain financial knowledge and awareness.

- Price the three exercise programs discussed in Chapter 8.

- Realize that not flipping carries a higher price tag than flipping.

6 "I Don't Have the Right Genes or Metabolism"

I had a client for over five years who constantly complained about her bad genes and slow metabolism. Three times a week as we exercised, I listened to her talk about eating healthy food and providing her family, many of whom were also overweight, with the same. One night I bumped into her and her family at a restaurant. I could see that she was uncomfortable. On the table, there was enough food for an army. Pasta, steak, big baked potatoes filled with sour cream and bacon bits, and every bread plate filled with bread and opened butter. I said hello and quickly moved on.

At our next session, she said, "I guess we do eat more than we should." To which I replied, "I understand. Now let's really get to work on your food." I never heard any more complaints about genes or metabolism.

> "LIFE CONSISTS NOT IN HOLDING GOOD CARDS, BUT IN PLAYING THOSE YOU HOLD WELL."
> —JOSH BILLINGS

Blaming your genes or a slow metabolism is a very common excuse. First, let's examine the roles genes and metabolism actually do play with regard to our body's weight.

What Genes Determine

Our genes are responsible for the majority of our physical characteristics like eye and hair color. Our genes determine whether we are tall or short, mesomorphic (strong muscular build), ectomorphic (thin muscular build), or endomorphic (in between). Genes also contribute to our longevity, intellect, and to some extent our immunity, or risk of certain diseases, such as high blood pressure, high cholesterol, diabetes, depression, and even alcoholism. Does this mean that our entire lives are completely mentally and physically predetermined at birth? Of course not. Scientists have long noted the significant role that behavior and environment play in determining who we are. Behavioral researchers have conclusively demonstrated that certain so-called predetermined diseases and even behavioral patterns can be drastically modified and in some instances eliminated by behavior and environment.

Think about this point. If you are currently a smoker, you certainly must realize that your chances of contracting lung cancer and emphysema are greatly increased. Stop smoking and the risk decreases. Moreover, if you are genetically predisposed to contract lung cancer, by not smoking you significantly decrease the odds that the genetic predisposition becomes a reality. Behavior can dramatically lessen the impact of a predisposition.

Genes Do Not Determine What You Eat and Whether You Exercise

No gene predetermines how much you eat or exercise. Eating and exercise are within your control. You determine them.

According to a special health and medicine section in the *Wall Street Journal,* "An imbalance between our genetic makeup and modern society leaves us vulnerable to all sorts of diseases." Our bodies were originally designed to incorporate a tremendous amount of activity from hunting and gathering to farming and fleeing predators. In our modern world, we don't physically move about nearly as much as we used to. This is attributable predominantly to the use of labor-saving devices such as cars and computers and the excessive watching of television (we don't even have to get up to change the channel anymore). We don't expend calories, or energy, as we once did. When was the last time you "stalked" your dinner? I'm not talking about roaming the aisles of Gristedes, Kroger, A&P, Jewel, Piggly Wiggly, Pavillion, Whole Foods, or rummaging through the shelves of your

GONE HUNTING?

refrigerator. It's possible that our bodies will eventually evolve to reflect our new environment (such evolution has occurred in the animal world more rapidly), but that's not going to do us much good in the early twenty-first century. Today, we no longer need to expend a great amount of energy to survive, but we continue to eat as if we do. Are we doomed? Of course not. You are not doomed by either your genes or your environment. You can override both the genetic predisposition and the consequences of labor-saving technology by being cognizant of the calories you consume each day and the energy you expend.

Memorize the following equation:

YOU ARE WHAT YOU EAT MINUS THE ENERGY YOU EXPEND

WHAT'S
KEPT *YOU*
FROM
FLIPPING?

104

BALANCE OF ENERGY EQUATION

ENERGY IN (CALORIES) − ENERGY OUT (METABOLISM AND ACTIVITY) = BODY WEIGHT

It's a simple mathematical reality. Stop for a moment and think about this equation. Dissect the components. I'm forty-one years old. What I presently weigh is a result of every calorie that I have consumed and every bit of energy I have expended, metabolically and physically. A calorie is a unit of energy. The only way energy can come into our body is through the calories we eat and drink. Note, I mentioned drink because in the next chapter I will cite evidence that points the finger at liquid calories as being one of the current causes of obesity among adults *and* children.

3,500 CALORIES = 1 POUND

Since a calorie is a unit of energy, how many calories equal one pound? The answer: 3,500. Please take a moment to understand this concept. Thirty-five hundred calories equal one pound; therefore, when you gain one pound, you have taken in 3,500 more calories than your body required. Similarly, when you lose one real pound (not a pound of water as I previously discussed), you will have expended 3,500 more calories than you consumed. Weight gain and weight loss are simple arithmetic.

The "Spill" That Sticks

Food, or energy, is necessary for the body to perform various activities and to ultimately survive. Let's use an automobile to illustrate this process. If you drive regularly, you fill the gas tank of your car with gasoline, or energy (the car's calories), so that it will operate. When you attempt to overfill your tank, or "top off" (which almost every gasoline pump urges you *not* to do), you spill, either all over yourself, your car, or both. The tank of the car will not take the additional fuel. It's full and has been designed to contain a specific quantity of gasoline, or liquid energy. Period. Unfortunately, unlike the car, the human body does not spill to prevent you from overfueling. Instead, it takes in the extra fuel and stores it as body fat. In other words, the body fat is the "spill" that sticks. If you are presently overweight, it means that you have essentially overfueled yourself. In other words, you have taken in more fuel—that is, energy or calories—than your body needs. The only way to expend that excess energy, or body fat, is to use it. In other words, *use it to lose it.*

"Use It to Lose It" Strategies

You can use the excess energy (body fat) by electing to follow one of two strategies—or both (which is my advice). First, you can consume fewer calories. If you start consuming fewer calories, or energy, but continue to perform the same daily activities, you will force your body to draw upon its stored supply of body fat for that energy. You will lose some weight. But, just so we are clear, classic dieting, or restricted calorie consumption, addresses only the first part of our energy equation; it will not continue to work by itself after a few months. Note that I said you would lose only *some* weight. If you are confused by this concept, turn to Chapter 8 for a detailed explanation on why dieting without exercise does not succeed over time.

Restricting calories, or "classic dieting," may be one method you employed in the past to lose weight. You decided to try one of the popular weight-loss diets that focused on eating alone and did not address exercise. As I will explain to you in Chapter 8, dieting alone without exercise is doomed to fail. The human body is too smart. Remember that: The human body is very, very smart. It will adapt to classic dieting and prevent you from losing any more weight. To lose additional weight and, most important, to maintain that weight loss, you must exercise. Consequently, I do not recommend that you attempt dieting by itself. It doesn't work.

The second option you have is to expend the stored energy (body fat) by burning additional calories through your metabolism and activity level. Ah, we finally come to that word *metabolism,* which is used by so many to explain and rationalize so much. What exactly constitutes metabolism, and what is its function? Metabolism is essentially a process by which calories (energy) are expended in maintaining the human body. This maintenance encompasses brain functioning, digestion, breathing, hair and nail growth, and cell regeneration, to name but a few of the functions of the human body that require some amount of energy, or calories, on a daily basis to survive.

Genes 25 Percent, Behavior 75 Percent

How much of your metabolism is determined by your genes? The answer is 25 percent. The other 75 percent is completely and utterly within your control. Let's review that one more time: Your present metabolism is only 25 percent attributable to your genes. The remaining 75 percent is determined by *you.*

Surprised? Start accepting this fact. I know, I know, right now you are saying, "That simply cannot be the case. My sisters and I are all overweight, as were our parents, so it must be our genes." I wish I could tell you that your assumption is true, but if your parents and sisters—your whole family—have struggled with their weight, then odds are behavior patterns have caused this to be the case. When was the last time you sat down with your sisters and really discussed your eating and exercise programs? When was the last time the three of you decided to take a walk rather than sit and have coffee and cookies together? What are your family holiday dinners like? Do you all pride yourself on being great cooks? Very possibly you are all great cooks, as were your parents, but that could be the problem. Just possibly, your family placed a great deal of emphasis on food. Did you celebrate over food? Did you reward with food? Are you repeating behavior patterns?

You may be surprised by your answers and observations. We all deny certain behavior. Sometimes reality is just too harsh and we selectively edit past and present recollections. Always remember, you and you alone are responsible for your behavior.

The Safe Excuse

Remember the anecdote at the start of this chapter about the client who constantly lamented her so-called bad genes and metabolism? She insisted that she and her family consumed healthy, low-calorie foods. What did I observe when I saw the family dining in a restaurant? Observe yourself and your family. What is really occurring? What foods do all of you most frequently consume? What is your family's relationship to food?

In the exercises in Chapter 1, I asked you to go back in time and think about the first impression you had of your body and your relationship to food. If you haven't shared that information with your family members, do so now. Quite possibly, they felt the same way, because, very early on, all of you were overeating or had an unhealthy relationship with food and exercise. Think about it honestly. Do you really believe your genes were to blame, or were you just looking for an excuse for your behavior? I realize that this is a harsh remark. I don't mean to badger you, but the only way you can successfully flip the switch is to be honest and realistic about your past and present behavior.

The genes-or-metabolism argument is a safe excuse. It enables you to justify your present situation: "It just has to be my genes or my metabolism that caused this weight gain. It's just not fair." It allows you to be a victim and therefore not responsible for your present body weight and health. But it's not a valid argument. You *can* lose weight. It *is* in your control. You are not a victim of your genes. What you are is a victim of your *behavior.* Your body weight is *not* predetermined by your genes. Your body weight is determined by your behavior.

CHECK OUT THE SIZE OF YOUR NEXT FAMILY DINNER

"I DON'T HAVE THE RIGHT GENES OR METABOLISM"

BODY WEIGHT IS DETERMINED BY BEHAVIOR

WHAT'S IN THE REFRIGERATOR?

According to Dr. Graham Casey at the Cleveland Clinic, "what you have in your refrigerator may be more important than what you have in your genes." I couldn't agree more.

You need to return to the first two chapters of this book, and you must start to believe that you can be a success at weight loss. You must practice visualization and learn to see that success in your mind's eye. If you can eliminate this barrier of not believing in yourself and overcome your inability to picture yourself as a winner, you will discover that weight loss is within your reach.

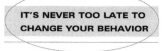

IT'S NEVER TOO LATE TO
CHANGE YOUR BEHAVIOR

WHAT'S
KEPT *YOU*
FROM
FLIPPING?

108

Behavior Prevails

It doesn't matter whether you are a Lifelong Struggler or a Slow Gainer; in both instances, *behavior* prevails. As a Lifelong Struggler, you were and are chronically overweight. Just because you started out heavy does not mean that you were predetermined to be that way. As a Slow Gainer who didn't have a weight problem for many years of your life, don't think that you are some sort of "genetic mutant" who suddenly changed as you got older. Quite the contrary. Your genes remained the same. What changed was *your behavior*. Your behavior caused your weight gain, *not* aging or some other factor such as menopause. Don't despair. You can change your behavior. At any age, at any time, you can lose weight and once again be in control of your body.

We're Busting at the Seams

Remember the statistics we discussed in Chapter 1? According to the Centers for Disease Control and Prevention, "we're not just getting fatter . . . we're getting fatter fast. The proportion of Americans who are overweight has jumped from 45 to over 64.5 percent and obesity has climbed from 12 to almost 30 percent since 1991." To further illustrate the point, "an estimated 17 million adults now have diabetes, up from nine million in 1991, and an additional 16 million have a condition scientists are calling pre-diabetes. Obesity raises the risk of diabetes tenfold for men, and an astonishing twentyfold for women. The percentage of children and adolescents who are obese has doubled in the last 20 years." This is not a result of our genes or metabolism; rather, it is a direct result of our behavior and society. Whether a Lifelong Struggler or a Slow Gainer, you are hardly alone in this struggle. You are not being singled out.

Our genetic makeup could not have changed in such a short period of time. Therefore, the genetic excuse simply cannot apply.

James Hill, Ph.D., director of the Center for Human Nutrition at the University of Colorado Health Sciences Center in Denver, says, "Why don't Americans perceive this problem? If these trends continue, within a few generations every American will be overweight." Dr. Frank Vinicor, director of the Centers for Disease Control and Prevention, adds, "These national increases have more to do with lifestyle than genetic makeup. It isn't our genes that have suddenly changed. What has changed is our society."

It is important that you start to pay attention to this development. Reread James Hill's comment. If Americans continue to gain weight at the pace they have these past few years, then within two generations, *every* American will be overweight. Genes? Metabolism? I don't think so. Don't become discouraged. All is not lost. You are not defeated. This is not impossible to reverse. Read on.

Exercise Can Trump Genetics

Exercise can be your salvation. The following bit of information will inspire you as you go about becoming a success at weight loss. Recent research indicates that exercise habits influence body weight as much as your genes do. "Being active can trump genetics when it comes to staying lean," says physician Lesley Campbell, the force behind this study. "Identical twins who exercise at a moderate pace carry six pounds less than the inactive twin; the vigorous exercisers can weigh twelve pounds less than their inactive twin." See what you can achieve with exercise? You can override your genes when it comes to weight loss. "Stick with it," says Campbell. "Exercise is an excellent way to overcome genetics."

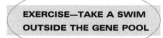
EXERCISE—TAKE A SWIM OUTSIDE THE GENE POOL

In my previous book, *The Business Plan for the Body*, I included a detailed analysis of metabolism and the additional factors that can influence it in Chapter 5, "The Financials." Only one variable continues to be the gold standard when it comes to boosting metabolism and burning additional calories, or energy, twenty-four hours a day, seven days a week, every day of the year. That gold standard is strength and resistance exercise. Yes, strength and resistance exercise positively affects a body's metabolism. Don't be concerned if at this point you don't fully grasp the contribution to increasing your metabolism that exercise makes. In Chapter 8, I provide you with a comprehensive explanation of that contribution.

PUTTING IT ALL TOGETHER TO FLIP

- The hand of cards you've been dealt is not as bad as you think.

- Strategic "card playing" contributes more to successful weight loss than genes.

- Successful flippers learn the Balance of Energy Equation and understand how to use it to achieve successful weight loss.

BALANCE OF ENERGY EQUATION

ENERGY IN (CALORIES) – ENERGY OUT (METABOLISM AND ACTIVITY) = BODY WEIGHT

- Behavior always overrides genes and leads to successfully swimming outside of one's gene pool.

7 "I Love to Eat"

I was at a party with a group of twenty people. One woman, at least one hundred pounds overweight, sat in the corner and pleasantly smiled. She never spoke. At the end of the evening, as dessert was served, the topic of conversation turned to something called a "chocolate bomb." Suddenly, this quiet, somewhat shy individual virtually came alive as she regaled the group with her past experience with "bombs," chocolate in addition to many others. On the way home in the car, I wondered how long it would take for my wife or friends to say something about this response. Well, it didn't take long. Immediately, my friend in the back-seat said, "Can you believe how that woman went on and on about the 'bomb'? I thought she was going to explode she was so excited!"

Who would have thought something like a chocolate "bomb" could elicit such a response?

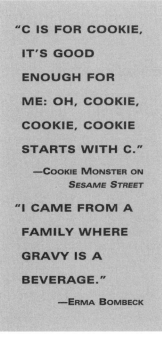

I understood her excitement. I love to eat. As an overweight child and adolescent, eating was my joy, my comfort, my sport (along with smoking). I looked forward to it each day. I still love to eat (but I no longer smoke). I learned to manage my eating to lose weight and ultimately maintain my present healthy weight. If I did it, so can you.

My goal in this chapter is for you to understand and accept two important points:

1. If you are overweight, you are overeating.

2. You *can* lose weight and continue to eat many of the foods you love—you simply need to consume them in a portion-controlled manner.

We Need an Eating Time-Out

Overeating is similar to a drug addiction, with food as the drug. All overweight individuals chronically overeat—day

"C IS FOR COOKIE, IT'S GOOD ENOUGH FOR ME: OH, COOKIE, COOKIE, COOKIE STARTS WITH C."
—COOKIE MONSTER ON *SESAME STREET*

"I CAME FROM A FAMILY WHERE GRAVY IS A BEVERAGE."
—ERMA BOMBECK

and night, 365 days a year, not just at Thanksgiving, birthdays, or other special events. Overeating becomes a compulsive behavior pattern and for many the centerpiece of their lives. Overweight Americans eat when they are happy, celebrating, sad, crying, in front of the television, at sporting events, standing up, sitting down, walking down the street, in a car, at an airport, in a social setting, in a private setting, during the holidays, before and after the holidays, on weekends and weekdays. Did I miss anything? As a society, we have become accustomed to eating, and then overeating, whether or not we are truly hungry or in need of food. Take a look at the following:

- Kelly Brownell, a psychologist at Yale University who studies behavior and obesity, states, "The number of opportunities to eat has risen dramatically. Food—usually junk food—is everywhere, in places people never thought one should eat—drugstores, gas stations, shopping malls and in institutions like schools."

- Restaurants and stores are competing for what the industry calls "share of stomach."

- The food industry currently produces 3,800 calories a day per person, far more than any man, woman, or child would need. Sure, some of those unneeded calories go to waste, but some do end up on our waist.

- In surveys where participants probably *underestimate* actual caloric intake, researchers have found that men, on average, consumed 216 more calories a day in the mid-1990s than they did in the late 1970s. For women, it was 112 additional calories per day. For the record, that equates to:

FOR MEN
216 EXTRA CALORIES × 365 DAYS IN A YEAR =
78,840 EXTRA CALORIES A YEAR

OR

78,840 EXTRA CALORIES ÷ 3,500 CALORIES (1 POUND) =
22.5 POUNDS OF WEIGHT GAIN A YEAR!

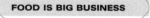

FOOD IS BIG BUSINESS

**WE UNDERESTIMATE
OUR CALORIES ON
A DAILY BASIS**

FOR WOMEN

**112 EXTRA CALORIES × 365 DAYS IN A YEAR =
40,880 EXTRA CALORIES A YEAR**

OR

**40,880 EXTRA CALORIES ÷ 3,500 CALORIES (1 POUND) =
11.6 POUNDS OF WEIGHT GAIN A YEAR!**

Consider this statistic for just one moment. For men, 216 additional calories a day equals 22.5 pounds of weight gain a year. For women, 112 additional calories a day equals more than 11.5 pounds of weight gain a year. *This is for one year!*

Consider the cumulative effect of this after three, four, or five years and realize that in the future the number of opportunities to consume food throughout the day will undoubtedly increase just as dramatically as calorie consumption has. Why? If you *continue* to consume more calories, the food companies will *continue* to make the food more available. The situation will *continue* to spiral out of control. Are you seeing this relationship?

Observe the Passing Parade— Adults *and* Children

One does not have to be in the weight-management business to have noticed the "plumping" of America. Do a little research on your own. Sit in a public place like an airport or a shopping mall and observe the passing scene. Sit there for fifteen minutes. What do you see? It seems as if every other individual is overweight—and not just a little overweight but considerably overweight. It's not only adults but children as well. Once again, I want to help you understand why this has taken place. Restaurants and stores are competing for what is called "share of stomach." Anyone who has ever studied or read about marketing knows that one of the goals of a marketing program is to increase market share (an item's percentage of the market—think of Coke's percentage of the overall soft drink market) in addition to increasing the overall demand for the product or service (increasing the overall consumption of all soda). Restaurants and food manufacturers want you to desire to eat more.

Plumping at the Pump

I have been driving for almost twenty-five years and remember when gas stations basically sold gasoline, related auto products, cigarettes, and perhaps soda. Today, gas stations are virtually grocery stores of junk food. Did you ever notice they rarely seem to carry fruits and vegetables? The choices tend to be buttered popcorn, which is prepared similar to movie-theater popcorn in tons of fat and is one of the most caloric foods available (a large popcorn is more than 1,600 calories, and it's not as large as you may like); candy; and huge containers you can fill with soda, cookies, cakes, and assorted salty snacks. All of these items are densely caloric. When you are at the pump, you'll notice that gas stations, in addition to strategically placed food courts in shopping malls, airports, ballparks, and retail stores, are designed to tempt you to eat, most likely when you aren't even hungry. Food, especially fatty fast food, is always being put in front of us. Ironically, you'll find a vast selection of fast-food franchises located within, of all places, hospitals.

Even Doughnuts Have Lobbyists

As if the proliferation of easily available fast food wasn't enough, consider the following quote from Dr. Marion Nestle, Ph.D., a professor and chairman of the Department of Nutrition and Food Studies at New York University: "There isn't a single food or nutrient that does not have its own lobbying group. These groups watch everything that the government does with intense scrutiny. Anything that indicates a government agency may say 'eat less,' they're right on top of it."

So, even the government seems powerless when it comes to curbing America's love affair with bountiful, readily available, high-calorie food. How do we manage these temptations? We begin right now. Remember, overeating is largely an addictive behavior, and the first step in breaking free of its hold is to examine why we originally developed this pattern. Just as I have urged you to do throughout this book, I want you to complete the following sentence to explore your initial relationship with food: *During my childhood, eating made me feel . . .* (Use the space provided on page 115.)

Here are my thoughts: *During my childhood, eating made me feel happy, especially certain foods. I loved ice cream, chips, candy, and tons*

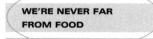

WE'RE NEVER FAR
FROM FOOD

of real buttered popcorn. When I was sick and home from school, only buttered toast with feta cheese gave me comfort. Food momentarily made me feel better, then I would look down at my potbelly and feel worse. Food never let me down, so I was always, always thinking about it.

Reading that today makes me sad. Okay, I didn't have a "Beaver Cleaver" childhood, but who really did? To drown out the noise of fighting, or to ease the persistent tension in my home when I was growing up, I ate. Simple. It is always interesting to me how many people have told me the same thing. From very early on, to mask or escape emotional pain, they ate. Some people have gone so far as to say that the only time they didn't feel pain was when they were chewing. And most of the time, they weren't chewing celery. What did you write regarding how you felt about food during your childhood? My guess is that you expressed similar sentiments.

Are You a User?

As you know, I am a Lifelong Struggler. I am a user of food. I have had to learn not to use food to comfort and ease emotional pain. Interestingly enough, I feel better today not turning to old habits, but it doesn't mean that I am fully "cured." None of us who have food issues is ever cured. We simply learn to manage better.

The Slow Gainer probably wrote a slightly different paragraph. Slow Gainers didn't have eating issues during childhood, but they are presently overeating. It's possible that their relationship with food changed as they progressed through life. Sometimes the food became an award for professional and personal accomplishments. Other times it might have served as a refuge from a hostile world as the years progressed.

"I LOVE TO EAT"

During my childhood, eating made me feel . . .

And, of course, there are those individuals who were simply unaware of their behavior until they had a physical exam, caught a glimpse of themselves in a photograph, or perhaps attended a school reunion. Keep in mind, weight gain is a relatively slow process, but a continual process. Whether you are a Slow Gainer or a Lifelong Struggler, understand and accept that if you are overweight, it is a result of your eating behavior and level of activity and metabolism. Yes, both groups are overeating for slightly different reasons, but that does not change the fact that both are overeating. Don't forget, your weight is determined by your behavior and how it applies to the Balance of Energy Equation.

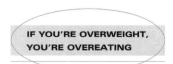

BALANCE OF ENERGY EQUATION

ENERGY IN (CALORIES) − ENERGY OUT (METABOLISM AND ACTIVITY) = BODY WEIGHT

If you are presently ten, twenty, thirty, or more pounds overweight and are "holding" at that weight, then you are continuing to overeat. If you decide to consume fewer calories, you would lose weight. This point is so significant that it warrants repeating. If you are overweight, you are continually overeating in order to maintain the excess weight. An individual does *not* stay overweight without overeating. Consider this in relation to the Balance of Energy Equation. Let's say your energy out (metabolism and activity) is a constant. Then, if your energy in, or calories, decreases, then your body weight would decrease. How can it not? Take a look at how to manipulate the variables.

If your weight is staying the same, then your equation is as follows:

ENERGY IN (SAME) − ENERGY OUT (SAME) = BODY WEIGHT STAYS THE SAME

If you elect to reduce your body weight by eating less, then your equation is as follows:

ENERGY IN (DOWN) − ENERGY OUT (SAME) = BODY WEIGHT GOES DOWN

In the next chapter, we will look at your third option, which is:

ENERGY IN (SAME) − ENERGY OUT (INCREASE) = BODY WEIGHT GOES DOWN

We're All Eating Experts

Of all the chapters in this book, this one is the most difficult for readers to come to terms with, even more so than the previous chapter, which discussed metabolism and genes. Why is this so? Everyone possesses preconceived notions regarding eating. We often behave as if we're experts on diet, primarily because we've absorbed so much information—much of it false—as we've "shopped" through the vast diet marketplace. For instance, many individuals don't think they are eating too much; some actually think they don't eat enough, or they're eating too many carbohydrates or too much protein. To better understand eating behavior, it is first necessary to separate *why* you are eating from *what* you are eating. In order to explore the *why* aspect of eating, I want you to complete the following sentence: *When I am eating, I feel . . .* (Use the space provided at right.)

Here is how I would complete the sentence today. Years ago my comments would have been significantly different: *When I am eating I feel great. I love food. I love to taste. I definitely love to crunch. I look forward to eating and often decide in advance what I am going to eat and when I am going to eat it.*

I did not say, "When I eat, I feel comfort." I no longer experience that feeling when I eat. I turn to other things or people, not food, for comfort. I did not say, "When I eat, it masks the pain." I no longer use food to minimize or eliminate emotional pain. Also notice that I did not say, "When I eat, I feel less stress." To be honest, I sometimes feel more stress when I sense that I am overeating. I did not say, "When I eat, I don't feel as lonely." Eating no longer is my "friend." For so many individuals struggling with their weight, overeating is not the issue. Overeating is the consequence of some other factor in their life.

EXERCISE 2

"I LOVE TO EAT"

When I am eating, I feel . . .

Look for the Flags

SEPARATE *WHAT YOU EAT FROM WHY*

Examine what you have written. Did you mention "comfort," "lessening of loneliness," "less emotional pain," "less stress," "friendship with food"? If your paragraph includes any of these flags, then it's imperative that you begin to realize that you are using food as a form of self-medication. Food can be a social experience, a shared activity to be enjoyed with others, and, of course, it provides us with the energy we need to maintain ourselves. But it is not a form of medication; using it as such is dangerous and can be the root of a weight problem.

It Isn't Enough to "Just Say No"

Overeating tends to be an emotional response to something. You are using eating to mask other issues in your life, just as alcoholics use alcohol, drug addicts use drugs (this includes prescription drugs), sex addicts use sex, compulsive gamblers use gambling, and shoppers shop, shop, shop. That's why just telling you to eat less would, quite honestly, be of little benefit to you. Nancy Reagan's "Just Say No to Drugs" slogan was well intentioned, but it overlooked the complexity of the problem. Like drug addiction, overeating is a complex problem for which there is no easy solution.

WHAT'S KEPT *YOU* FROM FLIPPING?

118

"Eat less, exercise more" is the correct advice, but not effective because it is too simplistic. It does not take into consideration the multitude of factors that prompt individuals to overeat. I want you to understand the *why* behind this behavior. Reach deep within yourself and ask, "*Why* am I eating so much?" If you can determine the reasons for your obsessive behavior, you are much more likely to be able to modify it.

Public versus Private Eating

A good way to begin would be to explore your public versus private eating. I can't tell you the number of individuals, predominantly women both overweight and at an appropriate weight, who eat little if anything in public. I have been seated at charity benefits and dinner parties next to overweight women who play with their food. They barely take a bite. It's 8:00 at night. These parties may not be over for hours, but that doesn't matter. They are in public. They feel they will be judged for what they eat; therefore, they elect to not eat. You and I both know that either on the way home or the moment they step inside they will binge. How could they not? They're starving!

I worked for a period of time with a young, attractive women with a serious eating disorder. She simply could not eat in public. She would starve herself all day, eat nothing, drink only Diet Coke or coffee, and then go home late at night (as she has a very demanding job) and eat everything, I mean everything, in sight. Most of it was salt and fat—chips, popcorn, crackers—and then she would shift to sugar and fat—cake, cookies, pie, and ice cream. The reason for this behavior? It turns out that her mother used to scrutinize every bite she put into her mouth. This caused such a fear of eating in public that this otherwise intelligent woman just could not do it. She could not attend a business meal or holiday function. She always had to arrive after the meal was served. Granted, this is an extreme case, but I have had numerous clients express to me a similar fear of eating in public or a fear of having their eating "discovered."

So what do people who don't eat in public do? Generally, they will hide food. I see it all the time. While I don't want to give away my trade secrets, I frequently check out clients' kitchen garbage cans so that I can see what is inside. The garbage tells a story and often gives me clues. Right there, after asking clients what they ate the previous day, I see what they *really* ate. I get the data that tells me I am dealing with someone who has strong emotional issues surround-

DINING AND DATING

It has been proved that most people, especially women, eat less on a date. The reason? Possibly they are trying to focus more on the person and the experience and less on the food. Or maybe they just aren't that hungry when they are "interested."

DO YOU FEAR HAVING YOUR EATING DISCOVERED?

ing eating. When I feel the time is right, I will attempt to get to the core of the problem.

Do You Need a "Sit-Down"?

First, I sit my client down and in a nonthreatening manner tell him or her, "We have been working together now for several weeks. You have not lost any weight. You have been great in our sessions, I see your body changing, but I don't see the scale going down. Something must be up with your food. I happened to notice on several occasions some empty boxes of cookies and cartons of ice cream." At that point, the client usually admits that, yes, he or she has been overeating. We talk about it and try to get to the root of the problem. From time to time I recommend some therapy with a professional who specializes in eating disorders.

As you explore why you overeat, please don't use one of the following answers that I have heard from people over the years:

- I eat so much because I have a higher taste for fats than most people.

- I eat so much because I need more fuel to keep me going throughout the day.

- I eat so much because I just like food more than most people.

- I eat so much because I have to for business.

- I eat so much because it is always there.

I ask you not to use these excuses because none of them is the real reason you are presently struggling with your weight. Remember, this book is about eliminating the excuses you have relied upon in the past.

WHAT'S IN YOUR GARBAGE CAN?

MAYBE YOU SHOULD TURN UP THE LIGHT

Studies have found that if you are concerned about your weight, dimmer lighting can lead to increased consumption. Why? Researchers believe that dim light reduces inhibitions, which leads to eating more. For people without eating issues, the lighting made no difference.

It's Called a What? A Diet?

Food is necessary to enable the human body to function properly. In many cultures, food is scarce. I recently saw Frank McCourt, the author of *Angela's Ashes* (a book I loved), on a television show talking about his childhood and hearing that people in America were actually dieting to lose weight. He commented that he didn't understand the concept as he spent almost his entire childhood in Ireland hungry and at times starving. Our bodies have not made us overweight. Our behavior has made us overweight.

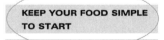

GET READY TO KICK
OFF THE FLIP

If Tom Can Do It, So Can You

One night I was flipping channels and came across the movie *Cast Away*. In it, Tom Hanks plays a plumpish Federal Express employee who survives a plane crash and ends up on an uninhabited tropical island. Because he has to hunt his own food and physically perform all the labor required to survive, he loses weight. In order to realistically depict the passage of time, production was halted for six months to enable Tom Hanks to shed weight to bring his physical appearance in line with his character's new environment and behavior. Clearly, his body had not made him overweight; his *behavior* had. The movie depicted this reality. You can do the same with your reality. It's your behavior. You control it.

In order to achieve a successful flip, I want you to follow the *Flip the Switch* Seven-Day Jump-Start Eating Plan, which I have outlined below. I've developed this plan over the years to help clients to begin dealing with the "energy in," or calories in, aspect of our Balance of Energy Equation. You'll consume approximately 1,200 to 1,400 calories a day. Yes, it is rather specific, but after years of experience I know it will produce results and motivate an *internal* flip of your switch. You'll find a shopping list on pages 125–126.

KEEP YOUR FOOD SIMPLE
TO START

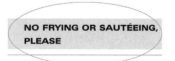

NO FRYING OR SAUTÉEING,
PLEASE

Flip the Switch Seven-Day Jump-Start Eating Plan

Take a few minutes to review the seven-day plan on pages 123–124. This is a strict plan and only a few substitutions are allowed. You can eat the same type of fruit each time a piece or serving of fruit is recommended. While a variety of fruits contain different vitamins and nutrients that are more beneficial to your body, for some people, keeping it simple at the start seems to work best. After seven days, more choices and variety will be added. For now, you can eat apples, oranges, pears, peaches, melons, and more when I recommend a serving of fruit. There is only one exception. I don't want you to eat only bananas, because they are lower in water content than most fruits. You should limit yourself to two bananas a week.

The same applies to vegetable servings. If you just love cucumber, then eat cucumber, or broccoli, cauliflower, green beans, peppers, asparagus (my personal favorite), and spinach (steamed, not sautéed— I had a client who lost more than ten pounds just by switching from sautéed spinach to steamed spinach; sautéed spinach is prepared with butter or oil, which makes it very high in calories). Be sure to always eat the portion listed each day on the plan.

You may substitute boneless, skinless chicken breast for turkey or vice versa. If you absolutely hate fish, then you may substitute turkey or chicken for the fish.

Go for the "Good" Fat

Certain fats, such as omega-3 fatty acids, which are found in many varieties of fish, are enormously beneficial to the body. Red meat is also allowed, but only once a week in the portion size listed. I am not anti–red meat; however, it is usually high in calories and saturated, or "bad" fat.

You may continue with the Seven-Day Jump-Start Eating Plan for as long as you like. This is a highly nutritious eating plan that incorporates many vegetables and fruits. After a period of time, you may decide to broaden your eating plan.

DAY 1

BREAKFAST: 1 packet instant oatmeal with ½ cup 2% milk, 2 tablespoons wheat germ, coffee or tea

SNACK: ½ cantaloupe

LUNCH: 1 can tuna packed in water, rinsed and drained; ⅓ bag (5 ounces) lettuce; 2 artichoke hearts; ½ cup tomatoes; 1 teaspoon capers; ½ cup cucumber; ½ red bell pepper; 2 tablespoons Just 2 Good! Salad Dressing

SNACK: ½ cup 2% cottage cheese

DINNER: 4 ounces grilled chicken, ⅓ bag (5 ounces) mixed greens, 2 artichoke hearts, 2 tablespoons Just 2 Good! Salad Dressing, 1 small baked potato, 1 teaspoon of Benocal Light, 1 pear

DAY 2

BREAKFAST: 2 frozen waffles with 1 teaspoon all fruit spread, 1 container nonfat yogurt, coffee or tea

SNACK: 1 apple

LUNCH: Chopped vegetable salad (mix the following all together): ⅓ bag (5 ounces) lettuce, ⅓ cup red cabbage, ½ cup spinach, ½ cup cucumber, ½ red onion, ⅓ cup broccoli, 2 tablespoons Just 2 Good! Salad Dressing, ½ cup 2% cottage cheese

SNACK: ½ bag baby carrots dipped in salsa

DINNER: 4 ounces grilled salmon, 4 steamed asparagus, 1 small baked sweet potato with 1 tablespoon Benocal Light

DAY 3

BREAKFAST: French toast: 2 slices bread, ¼ cup Egg Beaters, PAM cooking spray, ¼ cup syrup; coffee or tea

SNACK: ¾ cup frozen blueberries

LUNCH: 4 ounces grilled chicken, sliced; ⅓ bag (5 ounces) lettuce; 2 artichoke hearts; ½ cup tomatoes; 2 tablespoons Just 2 Good! Salad Dressing

SNACK: 1 container nonfat yogurt with 1 tablespoon wheat germ

DINNER: 4 ounces grilled halibut, ½ cup steamed broccoli with 1 tablespoon Benocal Light, ⅓ bag salad with ½ cup 2% cottage cheese, 1 nectarine

DAY 4

BREAKFAST: 1 packet instant oatmeal with ½ cup 2% milk, ¾ cup frozen blueberries, 2 tablespoons wheat germ (mix everything together and microwave for 90 seconds); coffee or tea

SNACK: 1 nectarine

LUNCH: 2 slices turkey, 2 slices toasted bread, 2 tablespoons Dijon mustard, ⅓ bag (5 ounces) lettuce, ½ cup tomatoes

SNACK: 1 apple

DINNER: 2 Boca Burgers on one English muffin, ½ cup tomatoes, ½ cup red onion, ½ cup 2% cottage cheese

---

DAY 5

BREAKFAST: 1 egg plus three egg whites, ½ cup chopped tomatoes, ½ cup chopped spinach (cook together as an omelet)

SNACK: 1 English muffin, 1 tablespoon Benecol Light, 1 teaspoon all fruit spread

LUNCH: Chef salad: 4 slices turkey; ⅓ bag (5 ounces) lettuce, ½ cup red cabbage, ½ cup spinach, ½ cup red onion, ½ cup red bell pepper, ½ cup tomatoes, 2 tablespoons Just 2 Good! Salad Dressing

SNACK: ½ bag baby carrots dipped in 2 tablespoons hummus

DINNER: Veggie burrito: 1 tortilla, ½ cup spinach, ⅓ bag lettuce, ½ cup tomatoes, ⅓ can chickpeas, ½ cup red onion, ½ cup red cabbage, 2 tablespoons salsa, ½ cup shredded fat-free shredded cheese

---

DAY 6

BREAKFAST: 2 slices toast, ½ cup 2% cottage cheese, 1 teaspoon all-fruit spread

SNACK: ½ cantaloupe

LUNCH: 1 can Healthy Choice fat-free soup; veggie tortilla: 1 tortilla, ⅓ bag (5 ounces) lettuce, ½ cup tomatoes, ½ cup cucumber, ⅓ can chickpeas, 2 tablespoons Just 2 Good! Salad Dressing

SNACK: 1 pear

DINNER; 4 ounces grilled beef tenderloin, 4 steamed asparagus with 1 teaspoon olive oil, ⅓ bag (5 ounces) mixed greens, 2 tablespoons Just 2 Good! Salad Dressing

---

DAY 7

BREAKFAST: 2 hard-boiled eggs, ¾ cup frozen blueberries

SNACK: 1 container nonfat plain yogurt

LUNCH: 1 baked potato, 2 tablespoons 2% cottage cheese, 4 tablespoons salsa, ⅓ bag (5 ounces) lettuce, 2 tablespoons Just 2 Good! Salad Dressing

SNACK: 1 nectarine

DINNER: Chicken taco: 4 ounces grilled chicken, ½ cup shredded red cabbage, 1 tortilla, ½ cup red onion, 2 tablespoons salsa, ½ cup shredded low-fat cheese

Flip the Switch Seven-Day Jump-Start Eating Plan Shopping List

Now I want to provide you with the shopping list that correlates with the eating plan. Once you have purchased all of these items, you will have everything you need to duplicate the eating plan. Check your refrigerator or pantry to see if you already have these items so that you don't need to overbuy or incur any unnecessary expense.

> **VEGGIES ARE THE KEY TO WEIGHT LOSS**

SHOPPING LIST

FRUITS AND VEGETABLES	QUANTITY	SERVINGS/PACK	CALORIES/SERVING*
Apple	2		120
Pear	1		98
Nectarine	2		67
Cantaloupe	1		29 / ½ cup
Asparagus (8 spears)	1		14 / 4 spears
Sweet potato	1		118 (5″ by 2″)
Baking potato	2		220 (5″ by 2″)
Lettuce or mixed greens (bag)†	4	3 servings	15 / ⅓ bag (5 ounces)
Spinach (bag)	1	3 servings	20 / ½ cup
Red cabbage	1		10 / ½ cup shredded
Red onion	1		10 / ½ cup
Baby carrots (bag)	2	5 servings	35 / 14 pieces
Broccoli florets (bag)	1		25 / ½ cup
Cherry tomatoes	2		19 / ½ cup
Cucumber	1		7 / ½ cup
Red bell pepper	1		13 / ½ cup
DAIRY/REFRIGERATOR CASE			
Benecol Light	1	1 container	45 / 1 tablespoon
2% milk	1	quart	120 / 1 cup
2% cottage cheese	1	24 oz.	90 / ½ cup
Egg Beaters	1	3-pack	30 / ¼ cup
Dannon Light'n Fit Creamy nonfat yogurt	1	4-pack	60 / 1 pack
Fat-free shredded cheese	1	1 bag	45 / ¼ cup
Athenos Original Hummus	1	7 oz.	60 / 2 tablespoons
Dozen eggs	1	1 carton	90 each

*Calories and servings are taken directly from food labels and from *The Complete Book of Food Counts* by Corinne T. Netzer (New York: Dell, 2000).

†Check the expiration date to ensure freshness.

Continues

GROCERIES	QUANTITY	SERVINGS/PACK	CALORIES/SERVING
Plain instant oatmeal	1	12 packets	100 / 1 packet
Wheat germ	1	26 servings	50 / 2 tablespoons
Pepperidge Farm Soft Oatmeal bread	1	18	60 / 1 slice
Thomas' Original English Muffins	1	4-pack	120 each
Fat-free flour tortilla	1	10	90 each
Knott's Berry Farm all fruit spread	1		18 / 1 teaspoon
PAM fat-free cooking spray	1		0
Cary's sugar-free syrup	1	12 oz.	30 / ¼ cup
Star-Kist tuna in water	1	3-pack (2.7 oz. each)	80 / 1 pack
Canned artichoke hearts	1	20 pieces	30 / 2 pieces
Capers	1		0
Dijon mustard	1		5 / 1 teaspoon
Healthy Choice fat-free soup	1	2 servings/can	220 / 1 can
Salsa	1	15/jar	15 / 2 tablespoons
Chickpeas	1	3 servings/can	110 / ⅓ can
Wish-Bone Just 2 Good! Salad Dressing	1		40 / 2 tablespoons
Olive oil	1		120 / tablespoon
MEAT/FISH			
Healthy Choice low-fat turkey	1	10 slices/pack	30 / 1 slice
Perdue boneless, skinless chicken breasts	1	3-pack	130 / 4 oz.
Halibut (4 oz.)	1		159 / 4 oz.
Salmon (4 oz.)	1		207 / 4 oz.
Top sirloin beef (4 oz.)	1		252 / 4 oz.
FROZEN			
Eggo frozen waffles	1	5	120 / 2 pieces
Boca Burgers	1	4	90 / 1 piece
Blueberries	2	2	70 / ¾ cup

Eating Rules

After you have completed the *Flip the Switch* Seven-Day Jump-Start Eating Plan (which, once again, you may stay on for as long as you like), there are some parameters I want you to follow.

Rule 1

Include a small amount of protein at each meal: breakfast, lunch, and dinner. Protein is the most difficult food to digest; therefore, it stays in the stomach longer, providing a feeling of fullness. Protein is a chain of amino acids. Many people assume that when you eat protein, it is immediately converted to usable human protein, but that is not true.

The Beaded Necklace

Think of protein as a beaded necklace, with the individual beads as the amino acids. What you take in as protein (the beaded necklace) must be broken apart into separate amino acids (break apart the necklace into individual beads) and then rebuilt as a new chain of amino acids to become human protein (restring the individual beads to form a new necklace). This process takes time, which is why protein is the most complicated food for the body to digest.

For protein at breakfast, I strongly recommend that you include egg whites (which really fill me up), soy breakfast patties, cottage cheese (go for the low-fat, 2% or less) or low-fat yogurt. Once again, if you eat a breakfast that includes some protein, you will stay full longer.

Rule 2

Eat at least five servings of vegetables or more each day. A serving of vegetables is equivalent to one cup, cut up, and is between 35 and 50 calories per serving. This requirement is easy to meet if for lunch or dinner you have a meal of a large salad with some protein on top. Or include a healthy portion of steamed or lightly stir-fried vegetables with each meal. You can even scramble some egg whites for breakfast

Unfortunately, many people shy away from fish because they don't know how to purchase and prepare it. When purchasing fish, immediately check for smell. Fresh fish should not have a strong fishy odor. I would love for you to give fish a try and expand your food horizons. Going to a restaurant is also a great way to introduce yourself to fish. Fish contains a great many beneficial vitamins, nutrients, and "good" fats (read on).

and include some chopped tomato, steamed spinach, broccoli, onions, or mushrooms. Vegetables are the key to weight loss, as they are high in fiber, high in water, and packed with vitamins. They also fill you up with minimal caloric damage.

In addition, scientists are learning to trick the stomach into feeling full. How? By consuming vegetables that are rich in fiber and water.

"Eat Your Vegetables": Why and How

I have had numerous people tell me over the years that they just don't like vegetables. If this is the case, give them a second try. It is possible that the first vegetables you were introduced to as a child were canned or overcooked (sorry, Mom). I had a girlfriend whose Mom, Betty, was a great cook (I still dream about her chili) with one exception: On Thanksgiving Day, she would put the turkey and the broccoli in at approximately the same time. The broccoli came out of the boiling water limp and a somewhat pathetic shade of light green. All of us begged her to wait until just before dinner was served to cook the veggies. We rarely won.

You may now find that fresh or frozen vegetables, properly prepared, are just delicious. If you have to, doctor them up. Here are a few ideas:

- Dip baby carrots or celery in salsa instead of high-calorie, high-fat, high-sodium chips.

- Steam spinach with garlic.

- Squeeze lemon or lime on everything. You can't go wrong when you take fresh or frozen vegetables and squeeze lots of fresh lemon or lime on top. Then take the leftover pieces of lemon or lime and toss them into a big pitcher of ice water. Everything tastes better and more refreshing.

PREPARE VEGETABLES
WITH CARE FOR
MAXIMUM FLAVOR

- Dip green or red peppers in low-calorie ranch dressing (I like the Kraft Free brand), or make your own dip with fat-free sour cream, a little horseradish, and some chopped onion or garlic. Season with great herbs such as tarragon, thyme, sage, or cumin. Experiment.

- Take a big head of cauliflower, place two pieces of low-calorie, low-fat cheese on the top, and wrap it in clear plastic wrap or a microwave-safe plastic bag. Microwave it until the cheese melts and the cauliflower is heated through. It is just delicious.

- Try different salad dressings. Avoid buying a whole bottle of dressing that you may not like by trying low-calorie dressings in individual packets available at most salad bars. (Don't be fooled by the words *fat-free*. Some of these dressings are still very high in calories, so read the labels.)

- Invest in a salad spinner so that with minimal dressing, you get maximum coverage. After you dry the salad greens in the spinner, add a small amount of dressing and spin again. You'll be amazed at how a little dressing goes a long way in the spinner.

- For lunch, take two pieces of low-calorie bread or pita bread (about 190 calories for the big pocket) and dress with Dijon mustard. Then add three to four ounces of turkey, white meat chicken, or tuna. Pile on sliced tomato, lettuce, cucumber, sprouts, or any veggies you choose. You won't believe it, but you could get two to three servings of your vegetables on your sandwich.

Eat Right: "Bright and Dark"

The brighter the color of the fruit or vegetable, the higher the amount of disease-fighting phytonutrients. It's the "orange" in oranges that may prevent heart disease and the "red" in strawberries that is packed with vitamins. So when you do pick your favorite fruits and vegetables, think bright. In addition to thinking bright, think dark. It's the dark "blue" in blueberries that may enhance brain function. Deep green spinach is packed with nutrients and vitamins; light green iceberg lettuce is basically water and fiber.

According to research at the University of Scranton, the cranberry

Try to add as much broccoli to your diet as possible. Many disease-fighting antioxidants are found in it, so eat up. Consider chopping it up and adding it to salads and egg-white omelets.

is the food with the highest number of disease-fighting substances. "Gram for gram, cranberries appear to be the absolute best food for fighting cancer, heart disease, and stroke," says Joe Vinson, Ph.D. Fresh and dried cranberries have the greatest protective powers, followed by cranberry sauce. Please avoid bottled cranberry juice, or drink it in very small quantities, since it is usually loaded with calories.

Rule 3

Eat at least three servings of fruit each day. A serving of fruit is one medium-size piece (visualize the size of a baseball) or one cup of cut-up fruit. The research about tricking your stomach into feeling full, which I just discussed with respect to vegetables, applies to fruits as well. Once again, this occurs because fruits are rich in fiber and water. Also, think as "bright" as you can when choosing fruits and definitely go with seasonal fruits when possible. If you stay in season, the cost of fresh fruit is affordable, if not a bargain (see Chapter 5, "'I Don't Have the Money'").

It is so easy to include three servings of fruit if you try the following:

- Start your day with a piece of fruit. Regardless of what you may decide upon for your entire breakfast, be sure to include one piece of fruit. This is doable even if you are on the go, since apples and pears are easy to carry and eat, as are bananas (though I want you to eat only two bananas each

COOL OFF WITH "COBBLER"

I love frozen fruit. Here is an idea. Buy a big bag of frozen peaches or cherries and put them in a microwave-safe bowl. Nuke them on HIGH for one to two minutes, add some low-calorie plain yogurt, and mix it up. It tastes like peach or cherry cobbler.

week, because they are lower in water than most other fruits). You may decide to eat fresh fruit with low-calorie yogurt on top for breakfast. That way, you get protein and calcium from the yogurt and a serving of fruit. You've just created a winning strategy to lose weight.

- Add some fruit to your favorite cereal. When I was little, I always wanted to have perfect strawberries fall on top of my cereal like they did on the cornflakes commercial. Those of you over thirty-five must remember that visual (how they kept the milk in the bowl I will never know). So start with a portion-controlled serving of cereal, some skim milk, and fresh berries on top. Once again, you get protein and calcium from the skim milk and a serving of fruit.

- Make fruit a snack. A friend shared this trick: Place fresh seedless grapes in the freezer and eat them as snacks or treats. Red or green grapes are both approximately 5 calories each for an average size. You have no idea how great they are when they are frozen. They taste like a major treat and give you a little crunch. Same goes for blueberries. Give it a try.

Rule 4

Always know the caloric value of "wheaty" carbohydrates. By "wheaty," I mean the bread, pasta, bagel, and rice group. I will touch upon this in more detail later in this chapter, but for now, just know that there is absolutely nothing wrong with these foods. What is wrong, however, is that Americans tend to overeat these foods. The amount of carbohydrates found in foods such as muffins, bagels, breads, and pasta has

"WHEATY" CARBS

FOOD	CALORIES
1 cup of plain pasta, cooked	160
1 cup of white rice, cooked	103
1 cup of brown rice, cooked	116
1 small piece of French bread (the size of a yo-yo)	80
1 small piece of focaccia bread	250
1 plain fresh bagel, such as Einstein's	500
1 plain frozen bagel, such as Lender's	170

exploded in recent years because of increased serving sizes, which increased the number of calories and subsequently causes weight gain. Therefore, you must exercise strict portion control with these foods and always know the associated caloric value.

Rule 5

Include a minimum of 600 milligrams of calcium each day. Scientists in Canada found that people who consumed more than 600 milligrams of calcium each day, roughly the amount in a cup of broccoli, a half-cup of cottage cheese, or a container of yogurt, had lower body fat than those who consumed less than 600 milligrams a day.

Robert Heaney, a calcium researcher at Creighton University in Omaha, made a startling observation. He notes that most women have a tendency to gain weight in their midsections in midlife, typically a half-pound to a pound each year. Those who consumed 1,000 to 1,300 milligrams of calcium from food (not supplements) had a weight gain of—zero!

Michael Zmetel, chairman of the Department of Nutrition at the University of Tennessee, believes there is a relationship between calcium and body fat because "a high-calcium diet suppresses calcitrol, a hormone that signals fat cells to make more fat and burn less fat." So, if you suppress the hormone, you will make less fat and burn more fat. Simple.

Bottom line, increase your calcium consumption in low-fat, low-calorie dairy. That is why my plan includes low-fat yogurt, low-fat cottage cheese, low-fat and low-calorie cheese, soy products, broccoli, and other foods high in calcium. Nutritionists generally recommend 1,000 milligrams of calcium per day for adults up to age fifty. See page 243 for more calcium guidelines.

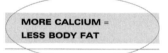
MORE CALCIUM =
LESS BODY FAT

I don't recommend that you regularly consume skim milk (with the exception of a little in your cereal) because it is a liquid calorie (see page 139).

Rule 6

Never skip meals. Eating breakfast is essential to your success at weight loss. Skipping any meal only leads to a diminished metabolism. Please, never, ever skip meals.

Eating breakfast may be the key to not just losing weight but keeping it off. Researchers from the Center for Human Nutrition at the University of Colorado Health Sciences Center in Denver looked at eating habits and weight loss in more than three thousand people. Of a group that lost over seventy pounds and kept it off (yes, that's seventy pounds, not seventeen) the study indicated that 78 percent reported eating breakfast each day while only 4 percent of the successful losers did not. The researchers believe that those who eat breakfast are better able to control their hunger and overall caloric intake throughout each day.

BREAKFAST-EATERS KEEP WEIGHT OFF

Rule 7

Drink plenty of water. I am going to make this as simple as possible: Before each meal or snack, you should drink eight ounces of water. It's so simple. Start each day with a big glass before breakfast, have another before each of your snacks and subsequent meals, and right there you have consumed between forty ounces (three meals and two snacks) and forty-eight ounces (three meals and three snacks) of water. It isn't difficult to add more water and stay properly hydrated.

The majority of people I work with who lose weight and keep it off continue to drink lots of water well after they reach their goals. They become water drinkers for life!

Doctor it up if you have to. Add lemon or lime. Drink bubbly water, such as Perrier or Le Croix, or flavored sodium-free seltzer, which I love. No, carbonation does not give you arthritis, as some people have incorrectly stated. And don't forget, tap water is just fine and free.

Here is another idea: Drink iced tea at lunch, then when you are halfway through, dump lots of additional ice into the glass. Do the same when you are drinking diet soda. Add lots of ice and watch your water consumption rise. Once again, just be careful: if these beverages contain caffeine, then they are also diuretics.

WATER TAKES THE EDGE OFF AND KEEPS HUNGER IN CHECK

I have one clever client who says that every time he starts to reach for something to eat, he first drinks a big glass of water. Frequently, he finds that he is not really hungry, just thirsty (I discussed this issue on page 85). Another client eats out frequently. He says that before he has any wine or alcohol, he drinks a big glass of water. He finds that he drinks less and feels much better in the morning.

Rule 8

Salad dressing and sauce on the side. Regular salad dressing is extremely caloric. I'll discuss olive oil later in this chapter, but for now, just note that it is 120 calories a tablespoon. Most salad dressings contain oil, mayonnaise, or some other fat-based item. A simple salad of greens, tomato, and carrots, probably no more than 70 to 80 calories, can quickly become a 500- to 800-calorie salad when you add the dressing. Restaurants love to gob salad dressing on salads. That's what makes them taste so good, but it is also what makes them so caloric. All dressing should be served on the side, and you should use it very, very sparingly.

Dress for Success

- Dip your fork lightly into the dressing and then into the salad—you'll use less dressing and you'll get plenty of flavor.

- Use about one-quarter of the dressing you are served. You'll find that it's enough, since most restaurants are very generous when they bring the dressing on the side.

- Skip the dressing and ask for fresh lemon to squeeze over your salad instead.

WHERE'S BRUTUS WHEN YOU NEED HIM?

For the record, Brutus did in Julius Caesar, but "Caesar" is doing you in as well—salad-wise, that is. Caesar salad is the most frequently ordered salad. Full of oil, cheese, croutons (which are fried in butter and full of calories), and egg, it is laden with fat and calories. A typical Caesar salad can be 600 to 800 calories. Many people have told me, virtuously, "I just had a chicken Caesar salad for lunch." I generally respond, "You would have been better off with a steak."

- Ask for balsamic vinegar and use as much as you like. Balsamic vinegar is only 10 calories a tablespoon—and has a zesty taste.

- Bring your own low-calorie dressing and use that instead of high-fat restaurant dressing.

When it comes to other sauces, the same rules apply. I can't tell you how many times I observe people order fish or chicken and then see the look on their faces when it arrives swimming in a rich sauce, butter, or oil. Ask very detailed questions when you order. Make sure to have all sauce placed on the side. You will find that you rarely use it and in the process save yourself hundreds of calories. If you are worried about navigating a restaurant's menu, I will give you clear directions later in this chapter.

Rule 9

Always sit down when eating. I heard this one when I was six years old and already struggling with my weight. Honestly, a family friend said to me one Thanksgiving, as I was eating standing up in the kitchen, "You wouldn't be so heavy if you'd just sit down when you eat."

Though I definitely do not have fond memories of that holiday moment, she was right. Ask yourself, "How often do I sit when I am eating?" I know what my answer used to be: never. I remember a routine from the 1980s where a comedienne said, "I have the answer for singles clubs—just a row of sinks so that we all could meet and eat over the sink. Isn't that what we all do at home?" Yes, and I do believe it is something we do alone more than with others.

So sit. Get out a plate. Don't eat out of the container (though my daughter Olivia and I sometimes do that for fun with ice cream). Put all the food you plan to eat on a plate and sit down. Take a deep breath, drink that big glass of water, then begin. You may find yourself consuming far less food.

How to Have Your Cake and Eat It, Too

The key to this program is balance and moderation. I would never ask you to completely eliminate one food group. That will only lead

In the July 15, 2002 issue, *Time* magazine published a cover story entitled "Should You Be a Vegetarian?" the day after the *New York Times Magazine* ran a cover story called "What If Fat Doesn't Make You Fat?" that supported the Atkins diet, which has been attacked since its publication. These two theories are confusing Americans more than ever. Let's take a moment to explore them both.

The Atkins diet says high protein–high fat is fine; carbohydrates are the killer, so avoid them and you'll lose weight. Atkins came up with this diet thirty years ago, and though a lot of people liked it and lost weight with it, the scientific community has long scorned it. That was until this buzz-inducing cover story in the *Times Magazine* shook up the diet world. The article said that Atkins's central insight—that carbohydrates stimulate an overproduction of insulin, which causes the body to crave more carbohydrates and store more calories (body fat)—was, essentially, correct. This has prompted a major debate. Now everyone is taking sides. And they're taking sides because they like to follow a school of thought. But I like to follow experience.

There is wisdom in the Atkins diet, and wisdom in the words of his critics. Atkins is right that protein is good for you; he's right that fat can be good for you; he's right that protein and fat are digested more slowly, and therefore give us all a more full feeling for a longer time after we've eaten. And he's right that certain carbohydrates can increase our insulin levels, which tends to make us crave even more carbohydrates—a kind of self-fulfilling prophecy. But—and this is an important *but*—you can get carried away on Atkins, and people do.

For instance, Atkins doesn't worry about how much fat you take in. In my experience that's silly. The jury is still out on the long-term effects of this eating plan in terms of heart disease and cancer. Plus, the human body needs vegetables and fruits because they are loaded with disease-fighting vitamins, fiber, and water. Why would individuals want to remove these items from their diet when they have been proven to guard us against myriad diseases, including colon cancer?

I am also not an advocate of an overly strict vegetarian diet (I am not an advocate of any kind of overly strict diet). Plus, it can be confusing to choose a type of vegetarianism, as there are about a half-dozen different classifications. In my opinion, many vegetarians simply overeat exactly the carbohydrates—bread, pasta, bagels, and potatoes—that Dr. Atkins shuns. Very few people I know are thin *and* strict vegetarians, and let's face it, this whole controversy is about getting lean.

So I advocate a position in the middle. Eat protein, especially lean protein, eat vegetables and fruits, and minimize the wheaty carbohydrates. Please cool it with the butter. Yes, if you consume huge quantities of bread, pasta, and bagels you will shoot your insulin levels up, but I am not talking about consuming huge quantities. I am talking about being smart. Bottom line, fat tastes good and keeps us full longer, but a little goes a long way. The same goes for carbohydrates; watch your portion sizes. Remember, the calorie is still king. Exercise common sense and follow a balanced eating plan.

you to crave that food group more than ever and most likely lead to an eating binge.

I have a very interesting client in New York who grew up in Santiago, Chile, in a household where lunch and dinner were five-course meals. Each meal was served formally, and every conceivable food was eaten, from cheese and vegetables to soup and meat and finally dessert. No single food group or high-calorie, high-fat item was eliminated. Each meal was always followed by a sweet. Not one member of her entire family had a weight problem. Think about it. You eat all the foods you love, but consume them in a portion-controlled manner and lose weight and maintain the weight loss. It sounds so easy, yet you and I know it is more difficult than that. We need to condition ourselves to eat less and that's why the mental exercises I have prescribed are so important to weight-loss success. It is that simple.

I have allocated 200 calories a day for your "treat." If this is cake, great; cookies, fine; chocolate, go for it. You should not feel deprived, but you should be knowledgeable regarding the caloric value of what you are eating. I do the following most days. I have some licorice, hard candy, baked chips or pretzels, frozen yogurt, or Gummi Bears, which I love. I also like the low-fat or fat-free puddings that are packaged in individual 100-calorie servings, because they are easy. I know I won't get in trouble with any of my "treats," since I allocated the calories for them into my plan. Sometimes, my "treat" is wine or, occasionally, a martini. So read your packaging and look closely at the calorie count. Don't be fooled. A piece of carrot cake at the Cheesecake Factory Restaurant is more than 1,400 calories! Approach your eating plan with your eyes open. It is an eating *plan,* so *plan.* Planning and awareness are your tools to successfully manage your eating—for life.

SAMPLE SNACK OPTIONS

SNACK	CALORIES
½ can Del Monte Lite fruit	60
6 almonds	160
1 Edy's frozen whole-fruit bar	80
Mott's Healthy Heart peach or berry cup	50
10 animal crackers	130
1 "sheet" of low-fat graham crackers (four small crackers)	55
2 tablespoons hummus with 14 baby carrots	85
1⅛-ounce bag Lay's Baked chips	130
1 200-calorie protein bar	200

We All Slip Up from Time to Time

As I said at the beginning of this chapter, I, too, love to eat, but I have learned to make better choices and eat in a more portion-controlled manner. I'm *aware*. I know how many calories I am eating so that I won't get into trouble. Sure, there are times of the year, such as birthdays, anniversaries, or other special occasions, when I will take in more calories than I should. I'm human, and though I like to believe I'm perfect and want others to believe I am, unfortunately I'm not. I'm like everyone else.

So if I overeat, the next day I cut back so that I do not gain weight. It takes approximately *forty-eight hours for the additional calories you have consumed to become stored body fat.* If you cut back for the next forty-eight hours or increase your exercise, you will not gain any weight, since you have caused the body to use those extra calories you consumed as fuel for the following days.

Write It Down: The Food Diary

The most important tool I can recommend to help you gain a better understanding of your eating patterns and the calories you consume on a daily basis is a food diary. Writing down what and when you eat will be the *most* important tool you use to consume fewer calories for two reasons.

First, the food diary creates awareness. It's there in black and white, exactly what you consumed in one day. In addition to writing down the foods, you will also estimate, to the best of your ability, the caloric value of each food. You'll also automatically increase your knowledge of calorie counts, once you get into the habit of keeping this record. By listing the food, the portion, the caloric value, and the time when it was consumed, you will have the necessary data to determine if you are eating for emotional reasons, if you are eating during stressful times, or if you are not planning your day and subsequently getting stuck in situations where good food choices aren't available. Or you may learn for the first time that you are just overeating. You may also discover that you are leaving too much time in between meals and therefore bingeing out of pure starvation at the next meal. By doing this you are creating awareness and knowledge. Both of these are cru-

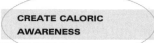
REGROUP AND ATTACK—
YOU'VE GOT 48 HOURS

WHAT'S
KEPT *YOU*
FROM
FLIPPING?

138

CREATE CALORIC
AWARENESS

cial to your weight-loss success and, if you think about it, apply to most aspects of your life as well.

Second, the food diary enables you to self-police. Since you know that you have to write down what you eat, frequently you will think twice about finishing off your child's fries, popping in a free sample of cheese at the grocery store, or polishing off the bowl of nuts during drinks at the bar. The diary causes you to think about what you are doing (managing behavior), just as the time-log journal in Chapter 3 caused you to look at the way you allocate your time and the budget in Chapter 5 compelled you to look at the way you spend your money.

I'm including a blank food diary page for your use in the back of the book (see page 311). If the layout isn't convenient for you, then by all means, modify it. I am also including a weekly meal planner that will help you with your food shopping each week. You will notice that the food diary and planner do not include fat grams, which have garnered so much attention in the past. Fat grams do not matter; the calorie count matters. Don't worry about the fat (though by no means does this mean to eat *all* fat); worry about the calories. Calories determine whether the body gains or loses weight.

Don't think you have to keep this food diary for the rest of your life. That's not realistic. I recommend to my clients that they keep a diary for the first few weeks they are flipping. Then we review it together, and I am able to give recommendations and suggestions that lead them to make healthier, "smart" calorie choices. Making better choices is a process. It's not something that happens overnight. As long as you are losing weight and feel that the diary is a positive force in your weight-loss program, then continue to keep it. If it starts to get tedious, then stop. Please understand, tedious or not, if you stop keeping the diary and your weight begins to creep up, then by all means start using it once again. Remember, a food diary is a positive tool to help you achieve your weight-loss goals.

Beware of the Liquid Calorie

One final point: I want you to include *everything* that you eat and drink, including water, in your food diary. Since we know that water is essential to the body, as I discussed in Chapter 4, I want to make sure that you document what you consume each day. Should you write down all liquid calories? Absolutely. Liquid calories are right up there with portion size as two top reasons why Americans have gained so much weight in the recent past.

I travel by plane a great deal for work, either promoting my books, giving lectures and workshops, or working with clients. Regardless of the time of day, 7:00 A.M. or 8:00 P.M., nearly 70 to 75 percent of my fellow passengers are drinking nondiet soda, fruit juice, or Bloody Mary mixer (which is full of sodium and calories) and alcohol. For the record, here are the calorie counts for these liquids:

LIQUID CALORIE COUNTS

Fruit juices	15 calories an ounce (120 calories per cup)
Bloody Mary mixer	5 calories an ounce (40 calories per 8-ounce bottle)
Nondiet soda	12 calories an ounce (144 calories in an average 12-ounce can)
Gatorade	8 calories an ounce (128 calories in a 16-ounce bottle)
Wine	25 calories an ounce (150 calories in a 6-ounce glass)
Gin, vodka, scotch, etc.	65 to 85 calories an ounce, depending on the alcohol content, and this is before a mixer is added

How do I handle flying? I ask for two cans of sparkling water with lemon or lime and call it a day. Okay, sometimes at night I do have some wine, but aren't we all human? I plan in advance to have some and budget it into my day. Even if I order wine, I drink as much water as I can get my hands on.

Big Slurp—Big Gulp—Big Calories

For years, most of my clients recorded their glasses of wine as four ounces. That seemed on the small side to me, so, we decided to call the glasses of wine five-ounce glasses. But the size of wineglasses has grown just as plate size has grown. You now have to allocate between six and eight ounces for every glass of wine. That equals 150 to 200 calories a glass. For women, who generally need to consume fewer calories than men, two glasses of wine can equal up to 400 calories. For those of you on a 1,200-calorie program, that equals one-third of your total! You have to constantly stay aware.

Tropical drinks, whether they are alcoholic or not, are loaded with calories. By drinking two mai tais or margaritas, you will have consumed almost 1,000 calories. Just be very careful when consuming tropical drinks. If anything arrives with an umbrella, beware.

BEWARE OF DRINKS BEARING UMBRELLAS

Liquid Calories Don't Quench the Hunger

The body does not register liquid calories the way it does solid food. Here is what researchers at Purdue University have noted regarding the body's response to liquid calories. In the study, Dr. Richard Mattes instructed one group of individuals to eat 450 calories of jelly beans each day; the other group was told to consume 450 calories of liquid, such as fruit juice. Both groups were asked to write down their total daily intake from all food and liquid. At the end of the study, it was revealed that the jelly-bean group reduced the amount of food they generally ate on a daily basis by approximately 450 calories. Why? Because the body signaled that it did not require as many calories as before since it was getting 450 calories of jelly beans, which gave these individuals a feeling of fullness, or satiety.

The liquid-calorie group experienced exactly the opposite effect. While they consumed 450 additional liquid calories each, they continued to eat the same amount as before. The body registered the 450 liquid calories, but these calories, unlike those of solid foods, did not tip satiety levels; that is, they did not create within the individual a feeling of fullness. The researchers concluded that the human body does not register liquid calories to make us feel full.

If you eat an orange, then your body starts to feel full; if you drink a glass of orange juice, your body feels nothing and wants more to eat. This study has provided an important piece of information for

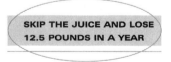

ONE CAN OF NON-DIET SODA A DAY CAN LEAD TO 10 POUNDS OF WEIGHT GAIN IN A YEAR

SKIP THE JUICE AND LOSE 12.5 POUNDS IN A YEAR

weight-loss strategists: Americans drink too many "designer" coffees, sodas, juices, alcoholic beverages, and other liquid calories. You need to become aware of the impact of this behavior and lower the amount of liquid calories you consume.

Recent research indicates that as childhood obesity rises so does the consumption of soda. Drinking just one can of soda a day could lead to more than ten pounds of weight gain in one year. Adults and children need to reduce, if not eliminate, their soda consumption.

Say No to Juice

How can I recommend that you say no to something natural, pure, fresh, and so healthy? Because juice is not healthy. Juice and "juice drinks" are full of calories and rarely provide any of the benefits, such as fiber, of the real whole fruit.

Children drink far too much juice, and parents need to be aware of this fact. I strongly urge my clients to stop drinking juice, and many of them claim that when they finally do stop drinking juice, the scale starts to go down.

You know I like to look at the "numbers" of weight loss. Say you drink one eight-ounce glass of orange juice a day. That equals 120 calories. Eliminate that glass of juice from your diet and guess how many pounds of fat you could lose in the next year—twelve and a half pounds! Taking juice out of your diet does not require a complex emotional reaction, though you may feel attached to that morning glass of OJ. It's just another simple step you can take to lose weight.

Eating Myths

There are so many misconceptions regarding eating issues. I would like to touch upon some of the principal eating myths and explain why they are just that, *myths*. Here are the ones I hear most often:

Myth 1: "I'm Really Not Consuming That Many Calories"

As I have pointed out, according to research, the average American male is eating 216 more calories each day and the average female is consuming 112 more calories each day than they did twenty years ago.

One of the reasons for this additional consumption is that Americans have become visually accustomed to a larger portion size on their plates. They seem oblivious to the fact that the larger portion equates to a greater number of calories. Many people are shocked when I tell them that they are simply eating too much food. They are truly not aware of the caloric value of what they are eating because they have become conditioned to consume these large amounts on a daily basis. What they see in front of them looks "right." My weight-loss management firm had a client who has struggled with her weight for several years. When she came to us for help, she was eating a very healthy diet. However, even healthy diets can contain too many calories. Once we got her caloric consumption under control, she began to lose weight. Her problem, similar to that of so many others, was essentially "portion distortion" and lack of awareness. To reverse this trend, homework and planning are necessary.

Recall the case of my client who was raised in Santiago, Chile. She and her family, none of whom were overweight, ate five-course European-style meals for lunch and dinner, including everything from meat to cheese to a sweet. Why weren't they overweight? What this underscores is the tremendous difference that exists between American and European portion sizes. *Self* magazine did a great piece on this subject. Here are some of the comparisons highlighted:

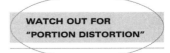

WATCH OUT FOR "PORTION DISTORTION"

EUROPEAN VERSUS AMERICAN PORTION SIZE AND CALORIC CONTENT

FOOD ITEM	EUROPEAN	AMERICAN
French croissant	2 ounces, 215 calories	4 ounces, 430 calories
Chocolate truffles	.25 ounce, 40 calories	1.5 ounces, 240 calories
Steak	8 ounces, 545 calories	20 ounces, 1,360 calories
Cappuccino	4.5 ounces, 50 calories	12 ounces, 140 calories

Do you notice how substantial the differences are? As Americans, we have become accustomed to eating larger and larger portions of virtually every food and drink. If we were to reduce those portion sizes, we would reduce our body size. John Travolta has said that he lost weight by eating all the foods he previously ate, but now he eats only half-portions—half a cheeseburger, half a bagel. It worked for him, and portion control can dramatically work for you, too. Go back to your Balance of Energy Equation. Reduce the energy in and body weight will go down. In addition to reduced portions, Europeans, and many thin Americans, observe a few simple eating rules. Read on.

Slow Down

Europeans eat much more slowly than most Americans. In Europe, the meal is a time to share friendship, thoughts, ideas. During a meal, the food is savored. What is the American approach to meals? I think the expression "beat the clock" sums it up pretty well. Let's face it, we originated the concept of fast food. Anything to get that food in a hurry, eat it in a hurry, rush, rush, rush, eat, eat, eat.

The European approach to eating contributes to a lower body weight. Why? The human body takes approximately twenty to thirty minutes to register that it is full. Americans eat so quickly that we are not allowing this mechanism to kick in and are subsequently consuming more calories than our bodies require. We are overriding the body's natural satiety mechanism. We feel stuffed after we eat because we did not give our bodies the opportunity to signal us that they were full. Had we listened to our bodies, we would have felt a gradual cessation of our hunger and would have consumed considerably fewer calories. American meals don't need to be five-course, two-hour events in order for us to lose weight. But, by slowing down at any meal, even a little bit, you can allow your body to help you with weight loss.

Don't Be a Big, Bad Wolfer

I am one of those fast eaters. For years, I would go to lunch with my business associate, Bob, and my former business manager, Patti (who is the model for my exercise programs in Chapter 8), both of whom

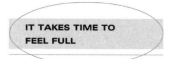

IT TAKES TIME TO FEEL FULL

I have a general rule when it comes to drinking wine. I drink two ounces of water for every ounce of wine. If I drink hard liquor, which I do rarely because it is so caloric, then I drink four ounces of water for every ounce of liquor. Why? Alcohol is extremely dehydrating. As you sleep, the alcohol breaks down and zaps a tremendous amount of your water supply. That is frequently why people who drink wake up with headaches. It isn't the alcohol as much as it is the dehydration that causes a hangover.

are thin and have never had a weight problem, though they each work out four to five times a week and do watch what they eat. The food would arrive, and I was nose to plate until almost all of my food was consumed. Bob and Patti would be talking, resting, eating a small bite, breathing, and irritating me immensely. I would get agitated and say, "Hurry up, hurry up, we have to get back to the office." Bob would say to me, "Listen, porky, we don't inhale our food like someone's going to snatch the forks out of our mouths. Relax!" (Bob is also my best friend, so he can get away with this comment.) It kills me to say this, but he was right. I've learned to slow down, and you can, too.

Draw Your Own Conclusion

When I observe a thin person eating, he or she is eating slowly. And every time I watch an overweight person eating, that individual generally is eating very quickly. Consider this another "Jim Karas Challenge." Watch your friends and family members eat. Who is eating slowly and who isn't? Most important, how quickly are *you* eating?

Here are two final lessons from the European style of eating.

Don't Eliminate Food Groups

Europeans, for the most part, do not eliminate food groups. Their diets include foods from all groups. Furthermore, most European food stores rarely carry low-fat or fat-free items. To Europeans, fat-free or low-fat items make little sense. If they want cheese (my personal pitfall—I believe most of us crave foods with either sugar or salt, and I'm a "salty"), they eat the real thing; if they want cookies, they eat the real thing. They do not eat large portions of these foods, but they enjoy each and every taste. I love that style of eating. I always find that when I have had dinner at a restaurant that serves a few different small dishes (I generally get two bites of each item), like a tapas bar, I always come away feeling satisfied but never stuffed. And, for the record, I don't gain weight. I am talking about eating five or six different small dishes, not sampling twenty-five different items, which is what many Americans do at a typical buffet.

Compare how Americans and Europeans eat cheese. After dinner and before the final dessert course, Europeans may consume a small amount of cheese, say the size of two dice (approximately ½ ounce). That is the cheese course. If you don't believe me, fly over to France and experience it yourself. Americans, on the other hand, generally serve cheese as an hors d'oeuvre, before dinner even starts, with cocktails. The American portion of cheese is generally a baked Brie the size of a steering wheel, along with crackers and other high-calorie items. Once again, this is *before* dinner. Do you see my point?

Watch the Snacking

Finally, Europeans rarely snack. Stop for a moment and consider what you consume on a daily basis between meals. Take a look at your food diary and you will see in black and white what and when you are eating. By minimizing or eliminating snacks, you will see your calories consumed drastically diminish. Don't be confused. As you saw in the *Flip the Switch* Seven-Day Jump-Start Eating Plan, I do recommend a small snack to maintain a feeling of fullness, but those snacks should be *small*, somewhere in the 100- to 150-calorie range, and should not be liquid calories. And, as I said earlier, please approach popular coffee drinks with caution. Regular brewed coffee with a little skim or low-fat milk and a small amount of sweetener or sugar is fine, just watch the calories in the milk and sugar.

Contrary to what many think, there are some positive effects to snacking. Research has demonstrated that eating small amounts more frequently can lower cholesterol by between 5 and 10 percent, so intelligent snacking may be the answer to both fending off hunger (and a potential binge) and reducing cholesterol. But once again, these snacks should be small.

IF YOU LIKE TO SNACK,
THINK SMALL

Calories Count

To enable you to obtain a better understanding of the number of calories in many foods and the appropriate portion size, I want you to begin to do the following:

Read Labels

Before purchasing a food or beverage item, it's very important to read the container label. Start with the number of calories per serving and the total number of servings per container. Multiply these numbers. That represents the total number of calories in the entire container.

CALORIES PER SERVING × SERVINGS PER CONTAINER = TOTAL CALORIES FOR THE ENTIRE CONTAINER

You then need to determine *your* average portion size. It probably is much, much more than you realize and greater than the serving size described on the label. That "small" bowl of fat-free frozen yogurt you've been downing may be more like 450 calories than the 150 calories you *thought* you were having. To better gauge portion/serving size, purchase a measuring cup, a food scale, and other items that establish portion size. If you go to my web site, www.jimkaras.com, you will find a complete listing of the items I am recommending and can purchase them directly. Here are a few visuals that should help you to begin to gauge portion size:

> 3 ounces of protein = the size and thickness of the palm of an average hand or the size of a deck of cards
>
> 1 ounce of cheese = the size of four dice
>
> 1 average-size piece of fruit = the size of a baseball or the size of an average fist

VISIT WWW.JIMKARAS.COM

You will also find a complete listing of calorie counts for popular foods on the site as well. Like the food diary, you don't need to use these for the rest of your life, just long enough to create or improve caloric awareness. Pretty soon determining portion size will become second nature. You'll quickly get a feel for what four ounces *looks* like.

As you begin this process, be aware that many of the foods Americans frequently consume are extremely caloric:

FOOD ITEM	CALORIES
1 ounce of granola	130
½ cup of premium ice cream	150–300
1 ounce of mixed nuts	160–180
1 medium-size fig	50
1 medium-size avocado	300
1 cup of guacamole	400
1 ounce of mozzarella cheese	90
1 ounce of Brie cheese	100
1 ounce of American cheese	110
2 tablespoons of peanut butter	190–210
1 tablespoon of mayonnaise	100
1 tablespoon of real salad dressing	45–85
½ ounce of croutons (about the size of two dice)	65

Diet Busters

I also want to mention what I refer to as "diet busters": traditional favorite foods that we may think of as being "healthy," when in reality they are loaded with calories and fat and can quickly sidetrack a weight-loss program. The list includes:

FOOD ITEM	CALORIES
Typical restaurant Caesar salad	660
Taco Salad from Taco Bell	850
Deli tuna fish sandwich	750
1 cup of hummus	440
1 ounce of pesto sauce (*only* 1 ounce)	150
Three-egg omelet with 2 ounces of cheese	600–700

Myth 2: "Carbohydrates Make You Fat"

Carbohydrates are one of the most demonized substances in the weight-loss marketplace. The numerous "experts" who espouse this myth in many bestselling diet books have many disciples. Here is the reality:

- Fact: Carbohydrates are the primary source of fuel for the body and, most important, the brain.

- Fact: All fruits and vegetables are carbohydrates.

- Fact: Current portion sizes of some of the most popular carbohydrates, such as bagels, pasta, and bread, have grown tremendously; therefore, caloric content has soared.

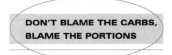

It definitely is not the carbohydrate itself that is causing Americans to gain weight; it is the *portion size* of certain carbohydrates. Reread pages 143–144 for my discussion of European versus American portion sizes. Never be concerned about eating fruits and vegetables; they should be the foundation of your eating plan. But if you are going to eat bread, pasta, bagels, and rice, you need to know the approximate caloric value of each. (See the "Wheaty" Carbs box on page 132.) Read labels, identify the portion size, and take a mental picture of that size so that you can make better estimates in your home and in restaurants. Ask yourself, "Are my bagels the size of yo-yos or tires?" If your answer is the latter, you may have discovered where some of your excess calories are coming from. Actually, yo-yos are smaller than most of today's bagels.

I'll Just Have a (Really Big) Brownie

In the original *Joy of Cooking,* there is a brownie recipe that makes thirty servings. In a recent revised edition, the same recipe, made with the same amount of ingredients, now yields sixteen servings. We are accustomed to our brownies now being about twice the size that they were twenty years ago. What happened? That's easy. Americans are used to bigger brownies, so the recipe stayed the same, but the portion size got bigger.

Myth 3: "You Should Stop Eating at a Certain Point in the Day"

This myth is completely contrary to how the human body wants to be fed. Digestion, as I explained, can account for approximately 10 to 15 percent of the body's metabolism, or daily calorie burning.

Skipping meals at any time of the day will only cause your metabolism to slow down and can play dangerous games with your blood sugar level. If you stop eating at, say, 7:00 P.M. and don't eat breakfast until 7:00 A.M., then you are starving your body for twelve hours a day. Your metabolism will slow down for half of each and every day because it senses that food is not readily available. It thinks that you are starving and will respond by decreasing your metabolism. So, not eating for long periods makes absolutely no sense. At the same time, as I mentioned in Chapter 4, abundant late-night eating is not good for anyone; in fact, abundant eating at *any time* is not good for anyone. But acceptable eating (a small snack), such as a piece of fruit, some yogurt, some cottage cheese, or even a portion-controlled serving of frozen yogurt or low-calorie ice cream, can be the smartest decision you make for your weight-loss program.

Curtailing eating by some arbitrary time each day is the same as skipping meals. Up to 60 percent of adults and 25 percent of children eat or drink nothing before leaving for work or school. Some studies show that skipping breakfast can *add* to weight gain because most people, adults and children alike, will reach for an unhealthy, high-calorie, high-fat "treat" in the middle of the morning to take the edge off of their hunger. They feel they deserve it since they skipped breakfast. The *American Journal of Clinical Nutrition* recently found that "eating breakfast may boost memory." That's just one more reason to stop for a moment and eat. Please don't believe that cutting off your food supply at some arbitrary time is going to make a difference in losing weight. It will harm you much more than help you. It's the amount of food you eat, not the time of day when you eat it, that matters.

Skipping meals forces your body to go into starvation mode. Therefore, when you finally do eat, your body is more apt to store the calories than expend them—you end up confusing your body. This is not a formula for success at weight loss.

Myth 4: "Olive Oil Is Healthy"

Not long ago, I was at lunch in New York City with one of my closest friends, Cynthia, and one of her friends from high school. Her

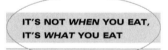
DON'T PLAY GAMES WITH YOUR METABOLISM

IT'S NOT *WHEN* YOU EAT, IT'S *WHAT* YOU EAT

friend is in her forties, attractive, intelligent, and affluent. We naturally spent a great deal of time talking about eating, exercise, and weight loss. As we were eating, Cynthia's friend was constantly dipping her bread in olive oil. Every time she broke off a piece of bread to eat, she first pressed it down into a plate to absorb the olive oil. After about ten minutes, I couldn't take it anymore. I grabbed her hand (mind you, we had just met) and said, "You *have* to stop!" She looked at me with big eyes and said, "What—what am I doing? Stop what?" "You have to stop it with the bread and the olive oil! Do you know that you have just eaten about five hundred calories?" I asked. "How can that be? I thought olive oil was healthy," she answered, clearly puzzled.

YOU WON'T LOSE WEIGHT BY DIPPING BREAD IN OLIVE OIL

Anyone who has heard me on this subject knows that I have very strong opinions regarding olive oil. Olive oil is 100 percent fat and 120 calories a tablespoon. One tablespoon! While it does not contain saturated, or "bad," fat, it is hugely caloric. If you must use oil, then olive oil is the wisest choice. But oil in general should not be an item you reach for without careful consideration. Okay, if you want to use *one* tablespoon to stir-fry a big bowl of vegetables, grilled chicken, or shrimp, great. If you want to spray *one* tablespoon of olive oil on a big bowl of vegetables in a salad, fine. If you want to sauté onions and garlic in a tiny bit of olive oil for a pot of vegetable stew or low-calorie chili, sure. You can eat some olive oil in the *Flip the Switch* Jump-Start Eating Plan, because it can make vegetables or a salad taste just great, but keep it to *one* tablespoon.

Dipping bread in olive oil is not going to contribute to weight loss in any way. Furthermore, eating grilled food prepared with tons of olive oil in a restaurant, whether it's fish, chicken, or vegetables, is not recommended. Restaurants use copious amounts of olive oil—have

Don't get caught up in the "no-" or "low-" cholesterol trap. So many people say to me, "Look, Jim, I'm eating this muffin—it's low-cholesterol"—as if that means it is also low in calories. "Low-cholesterol" claims are such a marketing sham. These products, including bagels and cookies, are loaded with calories. Don't be fooled. Read your labels and educate yourself about calories.

you ever noticed how grilled vegetables shine? Eating *anything* that profusely shines or glimmers, such as pasta salad, sautéed spinach, and many Chinese dishes (which don't use olive oil but still can be very greasy, usually because of peanut oil), is not advised. The glossy appearance indicates that the food is loaded with calories and will prevent you from losing weight. Remember this: Shine and glimmer mean lots of calories.

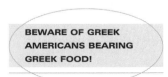

REMEMBER: SHINE AND GLIMMER WON'T MAKE YOU SLIMMER

Coconut and palm oil have 120 calories a tablespoon, are 100 percent fat, and are full of cholesterol. Olive oil is 120 calories a tablespoon and 100 percent fat. There is *no* difference in the calories between the two.

I always say the following: The difference between olive oil and most other high-cholesterol oils is like the difference between manslaughter and murder one. In one case (manslaughter) the person did not intend to kill, whereas in the other case (murder one) the crime was premeditated. Bottom line, the victim is dead. You can say the same about olive oil. The principal attribute of olive oil is that it does not contain cholesterol, but it has the same number of calories as any other oil. While lowering your cholesterol level is generally advised, it has no bearing on your ability to successfully flip. In fact, lowering your weight will contribute more to lowering your cholesterol level.

The Mediterranean Staple

One final point on the topic of olive oil: Many food publications describe it as being healthy and nutritious. It's generally referred to as a staple of the Mediterranean style of eating, which is centered around fresh fruits and vegetables, limited amounts of meat, chicken, and fish, and a lot of olive oil. I am Greek and grew up with some elements of this style of eating. The portions are generally small, at least in Greece. Unfortunately, portions served in my family were more American than Greek. Don't think the Greeks in Greece eat the way Americans do at their favorite Greek restaurants. In the United States, we eat all the bread in the bread basket and slather it with butter. Native Greeks rarely touch the bread. In the United States, we go for all the high-calorie treats, such as saganaki ("flaming" cheese), pastitsio (Greek lasagna), spanakopita (spinach pie—anything in phyllo dough is loaded with butter, calories, and fat), and the big desserts,

BEWARE OF GREEK AMERICANS BEARING GREEK FOOD!

such as baklava (the honey-dipped, sticky phyllo dough with nuts) and kourabiedes (sugar-coated cookies), my childhood favorite.

That is not the way Greeks in Greece do it. The Greeks eat lots of fresh fruits and vegetables; very small pieces of meat, chicken, or fish, prepared with reasonable amounts of olive oil (if prepared with oil at all); and a taste of dessert. If you don't believe me, hop on a plane and hang out on a Greek island for your next vacation. Watch the Greeks eat, not the tourists. Now, don't spend your entire vacation watching people eating—that's easy enough to do here. Nor should you feel compelled to eat since you are observing people eating. You'll be surprised. And by the way, in Greece, people walk to these restaurants. In the United States, we drive everywhere.

Myth 5: "I Don't Think I'm Eating Enough"

I have been in the weight-loss business for more than fifteen years and I have never encountered anyone, not a single individual, who was overweight because he or she underate. Yet, I am constantly approached by individuals who express this fear or who believe in the myth that they are not eating enough. None of them are thin. They are simply in denial about the amount of food they are eating and its caloric value, or they are unaware of what and how much they are consuming. (This is why the food diary is such an essential tool.)

If someone is truly not eating enough, then his or her physical appearance would reflect such behavior. That would make sense. The reality is, individuals who undereat are underweight. Individuals who are overweight are so because they overeat. Their Balance of Energy Equation is out of whack. Honestly count your calories and you will realize and see the truth. I promise. You're not undereating, you're overeating.

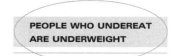

PEOPLE WHO UNDEREAT ARE UNDERWEIGHT

Myth 6: "Fat-Free Means Calorie-Free"

This belief could be the number one reason why Americans have gained so much weight in the past decade. I remember when fat-free products first became available. Supermarkets were sold out of these products in a matter of hours. (Hey, I was there buying up the

BIGGER PORTIONS, BIGGER PEOPLE

Researchers at New York University uncovered the following: The biggest increase in portion size happened in the 1980s and the 1990s, just when the increase in the size of Americans occurred. Surprise! Here are a few illustrations:

- Muffins used to be 1 ounce; now they are 6 to 11 ounces and anywhere from 350 to 800 calories.

- A serving of pasta was once 1 cup; now it is 3 to 4 cups.

- Cookies were ½ ounce; now they are 4 ounces and up to 400 calories each.

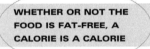

WHETHER OR NOT THE FOOD IS FAT-FREE, A CALORIE IS A CALORIE

Entenmann's fat-free pastries and eating the entire box.) Consumers rushed to grab the fat-free ice cream, cakes, cookies, and frozen yogurt with the deluded belief that fat-free equated to calorie-free. This can't be further from the truth.

What happened? People ate two, three, or four times the amount of the product (I ate the whole container) than they normally would have eaten because they believed, incorrectly, that by not eating fat they would not get fat. Return to your Balance of Energy Equation. Does it say, "If you eat too many *fat* calories, you will gain weight?" No. It says, "If you consume more calories than you expend, you will gain weight." *A calorie is a calorie.* You are not alone if you are confused by this point, but from now on, you will understand the distinction.

Next time you're in the supermarket, don't automatically reach for the fat-free item. Compare. If fat-free still appears to be the wiser choice, you now know that even fat-free can turn into your enemy (body fat) as you work to successfully flip the switch.

Fat Is Good

The low-fat or fat-free item often has the same number of calories as the original. Had you eaten one or two of the original, you would have saved yourself hundreds, perhaps thousands, of calories. This brings me to my final point. Fat, in food, does make one feel more full. It contributes to our physical and emotional "level of satisfaction." Fat is not the culprit in creating an overweight individual—calories are. Keep in mind that boneless, skinless chicken breast is

25 percent fat. Fish has fat. Salmon, which I love, is almost 50 percent fat. Even most fruits and vegetables contain some trace amount of fat (avocado, an exception, is 90 percent fat). Fat should be consumed. Fat is necessary to our health. To lose weight, you must consume fewer calories, not necessarily less fat.

Saturated, or so-called bad, fat is found in meat, cheese, eggs, and other such foods containing animal protein. This type of fat should be consumed in limited amounts to avoid the risk of certain diseases that have been directly linked to saturated fat intake, including heart disease and cancer. Remember, I am opposed to olive oil not because of its 100 percent fat content but because it is 120 calories per tablespoon and, unfortunately, a large percentage of Americans rarely limit themselves to one tablespoon of anything. Bear in mind, a tablespoonful is not a large amount. Check it out by pouring yourself a tablespoonful of your favorite olive oil; then pour it onto a plate and note the size. Surprised?

Myth 7: "Restaurant Food Won't Hurt My Diet"

Not true. Restaurant food, if ordered carelessly (also see page 65), can wreck your diet. In the past decade, restaurant portions have virtually exploded. Add to that the fact that you can't control how your food is prepared, and therefore you can't control calories. Before you eat out or order in, consider the following:

- The size of all plates used in most restaurants has increased. This includes appetizer plates, salad plates, bread plates, soup bowls, and entrée and dessert plates. The entrée plates alone have increased four inches in diameter.

SMART SNACKS

One piece of fruit = 100 calories

One 1-ounce bag of Lay's baked chips = 130 calories

One 8-ounce low-fat Dannon plain yogurt = 150 calories

½ cup of low-fat or 2 percent cottage cheese = 80–90 calories

One "sheet" of low-fat graham crackers (four small crackers) = 55 calories

14 baby carrots = 35 calories

FAT—WHETHER IT'S "GOOD" OR "BAD"— ISN'T THE VILLAIN; CALORIES ARE

- As plate inflation has occurred, so has portion inflation. Food is relatively cheap for a restaurant to provide. Their big cost is labor. So, to provide more food is relatively inexpensive. It's good marketing. Diners feel that they are receiving more value for the dollar.

- We have taken the restaurant "super-sized" portion and brought in into our home. We are used to seeing a larger portion; it seems "right." We have gotten comfortable with that mental picture and want to see it on our dinner tables.

- We eat out more than ever before in history. Recent statistics show that the average American eats one-third of his or her meals away from home, either in a restaurant, through takeout, or by ordering in. This percentage has risen dramatically in the past two decades, especially as more than two-thirds of women now work outside the home, there are more one-person households, disposable income has increased, and there is a greater availability of prepared food. Please note that "eating out" includes meals taken out, or delivered and then eaten at home.

- We tend to dramatically underestimate the number of calories in restaurant meals. Once again, this is because of olive oil, butter, and other fats added for taste and because of portion size.

- A University of Memphis study found that women who ate in restaurants consumed almost 300 more calories than those who dined at home.

Prepare for Battle

Here is the advice I give to my clients regarding restaurant dining and the purchase of prepared foods. Consider going to a restaurant the same as doing battle. It can quickly defeat your weight-loss campaign. The restaurant is your enemy. I know this may sound harsh, but you cannot allow a restaurant to take control of your meal; you have to take control. I know, some of you feel uncomfortable doing this. You're concerned you will appear finicky or difficult, or be a distraction to the other diners. But how can you believe in your ability to flip and not believe that you have the right to control what goes into your mouth?

I eat out about eight times a week for lunch and dinner. I scan the menu briefly and am usually looking for either fish, chicken, or a salad. I avoid all the items with sauce. When I place my order, I politely ask the waiter to please prepare grilled fish with minimal oil and please place my salad dressing on the side (two moves that save me about 500 calories). I generally request either balsamic vinegar or lemon for my salad dressing. Don't feel uncomfortable making such a request. You're not giving complicated or labor-intensive instructions to those who will be preparing your meal and almost all restaurants will be willing to accommodate your request. Frequently, I opt for fresh shrimp cocktail, steamed vegetables, and a plain baked potato. Another great choice is grilled chicken and a big salad of mesclun greens with balsamic vinegar. I am not trying to discourage you from enjoying a restaurant meal. I want you to be able to relax and eat foods that you like in a portion-controlled manner, make the best menu choices (or off-the-menu choices, if need be), and not sabotage your plan to flip.

ASK (NICELY) AND YOU SHALL RECEIVE

And remember: Chefs pour olive oil over everything. It is on the pasta before the sauce is placed on to keep the noodles from sticking; it is ladled on salad; it is aggressively brushed all over your grilled vegetables and fish. This will dramatically increase the number of calories you consume. To prevent this type of meal from arriving in front of you, here are a few tips, some of which apply if you're ordering takeout or buying prepared foods from a supermarket or deli:

Restaurant Ordering Tips

- *Be polite with the waiter.* Explain that you want your food prepared with very little oil and request that all dressing and any sauce should be placed on the side. Keep in mind, a smile really helps. Don't forget, you control the tip and a waiter realizes that as well. If your instructions are followed and you plan to return to the restaurant, make sure to show your appreciation with that tip.

- *Read the menu carefully.* Don't allow yourself to be rushed. Search out words such as *grilled, steamed, poached* (I find that there isn't much a chef can do to add calories to poached salmon, so that can be a good choice), and *baked.* Avoid anything fried, sautéed, or

BEING A GOOD TIPPER WILL MAKE YOU A SUCCESSFUL FLIPPER

breaded, or any unfamiliar preparation. If you are intimidated or have a question, ask. Most servers are more than willing to discuss the preparation with you and relay your questions to the chef.

- *Avoid soup.* I love soup, but most restaurant soup is loaded with fat, calories, and sodium. If you'd like soup at home, then prepare it with low-calorie, low-sodium chicken broth, vegetable broth, or bouillon cubes. Always be certain to use the low-sodium variety of these items. Add only those ingredients whose caloric content you know. If you prefer a prepared soup, then consider Healthy Choice, Pritikin, the low-fat, low-sodium versions of Progresso, or a similar low-calorie, low-sodium brand. Here is a recipe for one of my favorite homemade soups.

HEARTLAND STEW

Number of servings: 8

Calories per serving: 185

Preparation time: 2 hours

2 quarts vegetable stock

2 medium potatoes, cut into large chunks (I like them unpeeled, but you can peel if you like)

1 cup cooked pinto or kidney beans (if you use canned, then rinse them well)

2 medium tomatoes, diced into ½-inch chunks

½ pound carrots, peeled and cut into large chunks

2 parsnips, diced into ½-inch chunks (optional)

1 medium yellow onion, cut into ½-inch chunks

2 cups green cabbage, cut into large chunks and leaves separated

1 green bell pepper, cut into large pieces

2 6-ounce cans tomato paste

1½ teaspoons sage

1 bunch green onions, chopped (white and green parts)

salt and pepper to taste

Place all ingredients, except the green onions and salt and pepper, into a large stock-pot. Bring to a boil and simmer for 1 to 1½ hours, or until the desired thickness is reached. Add the chopped green onions. Season to taste and serve.

- *Remove the bread basket.* Keep the "temptation" off of the table and you will save yourself hundreds of calories. And don't even think of adding oil or butter to any bread at any time. It's a caloric nightmare. Nibbling on bread prior to a meal can add more than 500 calories *before* your appetizer arrives.

- *Have a Bite of dessert.* No, that's not a typo. Order a small dessert and share it with others. This is especially true if you are in a social setting where dessert is available. You sit there, with your decaf skim cappuccino, eyeballing your dinner partner's carrot cake. Don't torture yourself. Have one or two bites, then push it aside. You just had a "treat" but experienced minimal caloric damage. If you don't have the willpower to do this, try a mint or small cookie to satisfy your sweet craving. Many times, you will notice that restaurants automatically bring a little cookie or tiny piece of chocolate with after-dinner coffee. Ask.

- *Drink lots of water.* I know I covered this earlier, but you really need water to stay properly hydrated—even more so in a restaurant than at home. Restaurant food will always have more sodium; you should just accept that fact. Restaurant food is high in sodium to pump up the taste. Salt also can cause you to eat more (think about how you often can't get enough salty snacks once you start). And, please, don't automatically salt your food before tasting it. Most people do this out of habit. Lay off the salt shaker and drink as much water as possible.

You Don't Have to Give Up Fast Food

You definitely can eat fast food and flip. Once again, you simply have to know the calorie count of the fast

EAT THE GRAIN AND YOU MAY GAIN

Some of the highest-calorie breads are the so-called healthy multigrain breads, varieties such as seven-grain, multigrain, and hearty wheat. These breads, while tasty and chewy, include high-calorie nuts, seeds, and whole grains, which is why they are so high in fiber. They sound great but actually are very high in calories because of their density. The more dense the bread, the more caloric it tends to be. Avoid these breads. It may sound crazy, but from a caloric standpoint, you are better off many times with plain old white bread (or wheat bread without all the nuts, seeds, and grains). I know whole-grain and even rye are far healthier; however, white bread, though not as tasty or high in fiber, has been fortified with vitamins and minerals and is lower in calories. If you just have to have the "healthy" bread, then assign it a high caloric value, possibly as high as 200–300 calories a slice—again, success lies in the numbers. If you purchase a loaf of commercially made multigrain bread, read the label for calorie information.

foods you are eating and drink lots of water, as most fast-food items are heavily salted. Again, a few ordering tips:

Fast-Food Ordering Tips

- When in doubt regarding calorie count, go for the *smallest burger.* That usually contains the least number of calories. A small McDonald's hamburger without cheese or mayonnaise is only 280 calories.

- *Skip the cheese.* The cheese on the burger can increase the number of calories by at least 50 and frequently by more than 100.

- *Skip, or minimize, the fries.* The french fries in fast-food restaurants taste great because of the deep-frying in oil, which is packed with calories and "bad" fat. Fries are densely caloric, but if you have to have them, order the smallest portion available. A small order of fries at McDonald's is only 210 calories. The Super Size order is 610 calories. Big difference! And by the way, don't salt those fries.

- Be careful of the following items at McDonald's or similar fast-food restaurants:

  - Hotcakes with margarine and two small containers of syrup = 600 calories

  - Low-Fat Bran Muffin = 300 calories (more than a small burger!)

  - Butterfinger McFlurry = 620 calories

I used McDonald's as an example because their caloric information is readily available in a small pamphlet at each restaurant. If you go to McDonald's take a moment to read it. You can learn a lot regarding fast food in such a short period of time. You will acquire the ability to order a low-calorie fast-food meal. Most of the other national chains provide similar data as well, if not in their stores then often on their websites or through a customer relations department. And keep in mind, your caloric knowledge is always growing, so as time passes you will become more confident when faced with fast-food menus. We have probably all seen the Subway restaurant commercials touting their 297-calorie sandwich with 6 grams of fat. Many other restaurant chains are now doing the same and offering healthy, low-calorie options. You have the choice when you step up to any food counter. Remember, you, only you, are in control of what you put into your mouth. Being knowledgeable will make all your food choices that much easier.

DON'T EAT A "FAST" BREAKFAST

Almost all the breakfast items at fast-food restaurants are high in calories, fat, and sodium. It's hard to make a smart choice when none are available. Try to avoid the fast-food breakfast or at least minimize what you order.

PUTTING IT ALL TOGETHER TO FLIP

- Being overweight is the direct result of overeating. Your Balance of Energy Equation is out of balance—strive for balance.

- Overeating often has an emotional trigger. Don't use food to self-medicate.

- The *Flip the Switch* Seven-Day Jump-Start Eating Plan and shopping list will enable you to realign your Balance of Energy Equation.

- A food diary is necessary to create caloric and behavioral awareness. Without this awareness, your ability to succeed at weight loss is dramatically lessened.

- Food myths are exactly that—myths.

- Restaurant and carryout dining should not prevent you from successful flipping, if you arm yourself with accurate information and make good choices.

8 "I Hate to Exercise"

At a birthday party for a client, I sat beside an attractive woman in her fifties who was thirty to forty pounds overweight. She had seen me on *Good Morning America* and had read my book, *The Business Plan for the Body,* and a number of the articles I have written. We talked about what she was doing for exercise because she was expressing a desire to lose weight and work with one of my trainers. She told me, "I work out on the treadmill and do a little on the elliptical trainer for an hour total, about five times a week." "Don't you know that I recommend that you do very little cardiovascular exercise and instead perform strength and resistance exercise?" Her eyes welled up as she said, "I know, I know, but it frightens me to give up the cardio. For so many years I have believed that it was the key to weight loss. I'm scared to cut back and feel that I would gain even more weight." "Okay," I said, "let's make a deal. Starting tomorrow, you do it my way and only do cardio for a few minutes and the rest of the time I want you to perform strength and resistance exercise. I'm sending you a trainer three days a week for the next four weeks. If you don't lose weight, the training is on me."

Four weeks later she was down six pounds. Eight weeks later she was down a total of twelve pounds, and twelve weeks later she was down a full seventeen pounds. She looks and feels great. She just signed up her mother for the program.

> "WHENEVER I FEEL LIKE EXERCISE, I LIE DOWN UNTIL THE FEELING PASSES."
> —ANONYMOUS

Let's begin by clearly understanding exercise and its contribution to weight loss. Without exercise, specifically strength and resistance exercise, your ability to lose weight and keep that weight off will be next to impossible. I realize that many of you will find this statement difficult to accept, but it is correct. Why?

Do you remember our discussion of restricted-calorie eating, what I termed classic dieting? I stressed the fact that the human body is very smart. When you begin to restrict calories, as you do on a classic diet, your body acts as if you were stranded on a deserted island with a limited food supply. Your metabolism slows to keep you alive on less food, since the body believes that if it maintains its present metabolic level, you might die of starvation. This is what occurs every time you diet. It begins almost from the moment you go on the diet. Have you noticed that you tend to lose more weight at the beginning of a diet than at the end? That is, assuming you ever made it to the end. What happened? Well, the graph below will give you a clue.

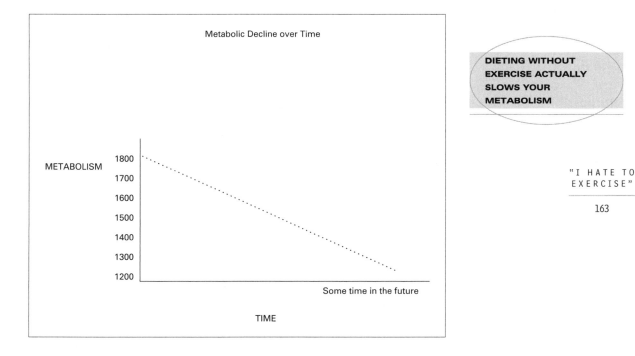

For purposes of the above graph, I assumed that when you began your diet, your body required around 1,800 calories a day to maintain its current weight. Then you began a 1,200-calorie diet. Over the next three months, your metabolism slowed to the point that you were taking in 1,200 calories and your body only *needed* 1,200 calories each day to survive. Applying this to the Balance of Energy Equation, at that point you were at metabolic equilibrium. Your energy in minus your energy out was equal and your body weight remained the same. If you have ever been in this frustrating situation, you probably said to yourself, "This is crazy. I eat so little yet can't manage to lose any more weight. Why is this happening to me?"

It's happening for a very simple reason. Your body learned to live on fewer calories each day. Consequently, unless you are willing to eat even fewer calories each day and every day, which I would *never* recommend, then you cannot lose any additional weight. And the moment you start eating more than 1,200 calories a day, you will begin to *gain* weight. Shocking, isn't it?

Here's the Answer

Now, don't throw out this book after reading the information above. No ranting. No weeping. Do not despair. Calm down. Relax. I have the *only* answer to how you can override the body's reaction to dieting. That answer is **strength and resistance exercise.** Strength and resistance exercise is the *only* form of exercise that boosts the body's metabolism twenty-four hours a day, seven days a week. Strength and resistance exercise is the *only* type of exercise that builds lean muscle tissue. It is that lean muscle that enables the body's metabolism to stay at its original levels and even *increase.* That's right, the way to *increase* your metabolism is to perform strength and resistance exercises.

You may have been wondering how the body managed to slow its metabolism when you went on a diet. This is an interesting and significant component of this analysis. This slowing occurred as the body attacked its most active tissue, muscle. By active, I mean the tissue of the body that requires the most calories on a daily basis to survive. Once again, that tissue is muscle, the most metabolically active tissue of the body. You operated on less and less lean muscle tissue, in other words less *active* tissue, which slowed your metabolism.

Muscle requires more energy, or calories, than any other type of body tissue (including fat) twenty-four hours a day, seven days a week. Each and every person, no matter his or her age, sex, or color, should adopt one principal strategy when it comes to weight loss—maintaining and building lean muscle tissue. This principle is so important that it's worth repeating: The key to weight loss is to maintain and increase your body's lean muscle tissue.

Why Does Muscle Burn More Calories?

By performing strength and resistance exercises, you're asking the muscles of the body to go beyond their present ability. First, those muscles start to fatigue, then ultimately fail in their ability to complete the exercise (more on this later in the chapter). As you challenge your muscles, you create tiny tears in the muscle fiber. Don't be frightened or think that this is bad for the body. On the contrary, this is what strength and resistance exercise is all about. These tears need to repair over the next twenty-four to forty-eight hours. As they repair, the muscle grows slightly larger. It grows because, remember, the human body is very smart. It says to itself, "If my muscles have to perform this exercise again, I want to be able to do it better." This whole process of breaking down and repairing lean muscle tissue requires calories, a great many calories. Experts tell us that one pound of lean muscle tissue requires between 35 and 50 calories per pound per day to maintain itself. Look at this analysis of adding lean muscle tissue and what it can contribute to a weight-loss program.

MAINTAIN AND BUILD
LEAN MUSCLE TISSUE
TO LOSE WEIGHT

**EFFECTS OF ADDING ONE POUND OF MUSCLE
TO YOUR PRESENT BODY**

ONE POUND OF MUSCLE BURNS BETWEEN 35 AND 50 CALORIES
PER POUND PER DAY

50 CALORIES × 365 DAYS IN THE YEAR =
18,250 CALORIES BURNED EACH YEAR

18,250 CALORIES BURNED ÷ 3,500 CALORIES (ONE POUND) =
5.2 POUNDS OF FAT BURNED EACH YEAR
FROM ONE POUND OF MUSCLE

**EFFECTS OF ADDING FIVE POUNDS OF MUSCLE
TO YOUR PRESENT BODY**

FIVE POUNDS OF MUSCLE BURNS APPROXIMATELY
250 CALORIES PER DAY

250 CALORIES × 365 DAYS IN THE YEAR =
91,250 CALORIES BURNED EACH YEAR

91,250 CALORIES BURNED ÷ 3,500 CALORIES (ONE POUND) =
<u>26 POUNDS</u> OF FAT BURNED EACH YEAR
FROM FIVE POUNDS OF MUSCLE

Or on a Percentage Basis . . .

You can also examine the increase in your metabolism on a percentage basis. These are significant numbers and you don't have to exercise every day to achieve these benefits. A recent study done at the University of Maryland showed that performing strength and resistance exercise raised resting metabolic rates by about 7 percent while other studies have show that metabolism may increase as much as 15 percent. These calories are burned simply by the process of breaking down and repairing the muscle tissue. Adding lean muscle tissue to the body will enable you to lose ten, twenty, even thirty pounds or more each year. And you thought you had to get on a treadmill and run ten thousand miles a day! You obviously do not.

Once again, here is the balance of energy equation:

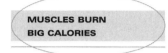
MUSCLES BURN
BIG CALORIES

BALANCE OF ENERGY EQUATION

| ENERGY IN | (CALORIES) − | ENERGY OUT | (METABOLISM AND ACTIVITY) = | BODY WEIGHT |

Manipulating the Equation

Recall my analysis of how you can manipulate this equation from Chapter 7.

If your weight is staying the same, then this is your equation:

| ENERGY IN | (SAME) − | ENERGY OUT | (SAME) = | BODY WEIGHT | STAYS THE SAME

If you elect to reduce your body weight by eating less, then your equation would be:

| ENERGY IN | (DOWN) − | ENERGY OUT | (SAME) = | BODY WEIGHT | GOES DOWN

In this chapter, we will look at your third option, which is:

| ENERGY IN | (SAME) − | ENERGY OUT | (INCREASE) = | BODY WEIGHT | GOES DOWN

But my recommendation is to approach both sides of the equation as follows:

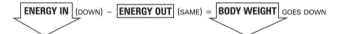

| ENERGY IN | (DOWN) − | ENERGY OUT | (INCREASE) = | BODY WEIGHT | GOES DOWN

If you opt for a classic diet approach, such as equation two above, then in the beginning, if your energy *in* is less and your energy *out* remains the same, your body weight will go *down*. But—and this fact is the main point you need to grasp—in a very short period of time, your energy *out,* which is the number of calories burned by your metabolism and activity, will go *down* because the body's metabolism will slow to keep you alive. Look at the new equation:

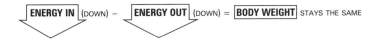

$$\text{ENERGY IN (DOWN)} - \text{ENERGY OUT (DOWN)} = \text{BODY WEIGHT STAYS THE SAME}$$

How does the body accomplish this? By devouring lean muscle tissue, which requires many calories daily to survive. Classic dieting achieves the *opposite* of what will enable you to lose the weight and, more important, keep that weight off and stay flipped for life.

DON'T ATTACK LEAN MUSCLE THROUGH CLASSIC DIETING

Look a Little Closer

Current scientific study takes this analysis one step further. Rescarchers divided participants into three groups to analyze how their metabolisms responded to three different scenarios:

- Group 1 restricted calories—no exercise

- Group 2 restricted calories—performed cardiovascular exercise

- Group 3 restricted calories—performed strength and resistance exercise

Both groups 1 and 2 experienced a decrease in lean muscle tissue and metabolism. Group 3, those who restricted their calories *and* performed strength and resistance exercises, saw their metabolism *increase.* This is an impressive piece of data that explains clearly which weight-loss strategy will succeed. Remember it and tell others who complain that they can't lose weight or that diets don't work. Yes, they *can* lose weight and diets *do* work. What is necessary to make them work is the inclusion of strength and resistance exercise.

DIETING DOES WORK IF COMBINED WITH STRENGTH AND RESISTANCE EXERCISE

I thought so. Researchers at Tufts University compared women on identical eating plans. The women who performed strength and resistance exercise lost 44 percent more body *fat* than the women who only dieted. No, I am not mistaken. Forty-four percent more body fat *loss* for the women who performed strength and resistance exercise!

Why You Hate to Exercise

According to exercise psychologist William P. Morgan, of the University of Wisconsin–Madison, "half of exercisers ditch a new fitness program within eight weeks, and another 25 percent quit within a year." I believe the numbers may actually be even higher than that. From my experience, people frequently quit exercise for the following reasons:

- *It just takes too much time.* Most people who embark upon an exercise program feel that they have to do at least forty-five minutes to an hour, five to six days a week, to derive the benefits of exercise. This is untrue and possibly even counterproductive. An individual can achieve tremendous benefits, as I will soon show you, performing strength and resistance exercise three times a week for thirty minutes or less. Don't aim to exercise long, aim to exercise smart. Exercise intelligently and you will produce results.

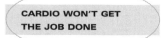
CARDIO WON'T GET THE JOB DONE

- *I don't see results.* This is absolutely true. Most people who embark upon an exercise program perform cardiovascular exercise. Once again, cardio isn't the answer to weight loss. Unfortunately, so many individuals walk or jog outside or go to their health club or gym, diligently performing cardiovascular exercise and unfortunately seeing no results. Understandably they become discouraged and give up. In a recent study, the National Sporting Goods Association reported that 81 million people in the United States participated in exercise by walking. Swimming, with 59 million participants, was second. Then came fishing, camping, cardiovascular exercise on equipment, bicycle riding, bowling, billiards/pool, basketball, and aerobics. Where was weight lifting? Number 11, with 26.6 million participants. Hundreds of millions of people performing some sort of cardiovascular activity (mind you, billiards/pool is part of that group), and our population is only getting larger and larger. And keep in mind, the majority didn't stay with their exercise program longer than eight weeks.

My goal is for you to see and feel the benefits of your hard work. That's what strength and resistance exercise provides. Within a few weeks you will see a "new" you right before your very eyes.

EXERCISE SMART, NOT LONG

- *I get injured.* Unfortunately, many people who begin an exercise program get hurt. Frequently this results from overuse, which is common among individuals who perform too much cardiovascular exercise (think excessive running) or simply were pushing themselves too hard, which resulted in an injury. My goal is for you to approach your exercise program with knowledge, intelligence, and a good dose of common sense. I don't want you to hurt your body. I want you to enhance your body.

- *I believe that exercise allows me to eat more.* I see and hear this all the time. I remember when I started teaching aerobics classes back in 1987 (yes, I, too, was under the delusion that cardio was the way to succeed at weight loss). After I taught not one but two one-hour classes (What was I thinking? My knees hurt so much I lived on aspirin), a group of us used to go out for breakfast. I would watch this group of predominantly women and a few men chow down pancakes, waffles, sausage, bacon, eggs, you name it. All felt virtuous because they had worked out. Mind you, almost everyone was overweight and wondering why. Today, I know why. They were eating many more calories than they had expended during the exercise class. They would have been better off skipping the exercise and just eating a normal breakfast. After a while, I noticed many of these people dropping out of class. When I bumped into one woman at a store a few months later, I asked her why she had stopped taking my class. She said, "All that effort and I never lost any weight. So I figured, why keep going?" I should have told her what she was doing wrong, but I didn't want to risk offending her. Today, I don't want to offend you either, but I do want you to understand that you cannot eat anything you like just because you exercise. On the contrary, the perfect time to couple low-calorie

DON'T EXERCISE TO EAT

eating with exercise is when you are performing strength and resistance exercise. You will really see results. It's motivating. It's exciting. For the first time, it's working!

Why Do You Think So Few People Succeed at Weight Loss?

Think about that for a moment. Think about all your friends, family members, and acquaintances. How many have lost weight and kept the weight off? Unfortunately, very few. The only ones who have kept the weight off are the ones who are performing strength and resistance exercise. Do you even know anyone who has combined strength and resistance exercise with his or her diet program? Have your family, friends, or acquaintances tried this approach? Rarely does anyone do so. In all my years of working with clients, the *only* people I know who successfully lost weight and who have kept the weight off are the individuals who continue to perform strength and resistance exercise.

Bear in mind that I have spent more than fifteen years in the weight-loss industry and this observation isn't a casual one. It's based on working with several thousand individuals. I cannot stress enough that successful weight loss occurred in those people who combined low-calorie eating with strength and resistance exercise. In other words, this is the equation that works:

THE SUCCESS-PRODUCING EQUATION

⬇ ⬆

|ENERGY IN| (DOWN) − |ENERGY OUT| (INCREASE)

THROUGH STRENGTH AND RESISTANCE EXERCISE =

⬇

|BODY WEIGHT| GOES DOWN—PERMANENTLY!

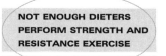

NOT ENOUGH DIETERS PERFORM STRENGTH AND RESISTANCE EXERCISE

Don't Be an Unhealthy Loser

Actually, there is one small exception. There are individuals who have lost weight but take an unhealthy approach to exercise. They perform cardiovascular exercise for several hours, if not more, each and every day. I have seen these individuals in health clubs and parks over the years, sometimes two or three times on the same day. You have probably noticed them as well. Every time you open your drapes or raise your shades the first thing in the morning, they are running by. Later, as you open the front door to get your newspaper, they trot past again. You eat breakfast, make a few phone calls, finish the paper, get in your car, turn out of your driveway, and almost hit them as they again pass by. Eight hours later you come home from work and, yes, unbelievable though it seems, they are at it again, now wearing their safety reflective clothing. What is this all about? These people are using exercise and body weight to mask other issues in their lives. This is by no means what I want for you. Excessive exercise is as damaging to your body and health as excessive weight, excessive drinking, excessive smoking—excessive anything.

THERE THEY GO AGAIN!

Throw Out the Treadmill!

Back in May 2001, When I was on ABC's *Good Morning America,* I said to Diane Sawyer, who lost more than twenty-five pounds on my plan, "The key to weight loss is strength and resistance exercise. Throw out the treadmill." My e-mail and ABC's e-mail were overwhelmed with people exclaiming, "How can this be? I was always told that cardiovascular exercise was the key to weight loss." Well, that has been the advice given by fitness trainers for years. They were mistaken.

TOO MUCH CARDIO CAN DAMAGE THE BODY

Today, we have amassed considerable data conclusively demonstrating that it is strength and resistance exercise combined with low-calorie eating that produces successful weight loss *and* keeps that weight off. This is the formula I have used with my clients, and the results have been spectacular. And these individuals have not turned into "weight-loss yo-yos" stuck in a vicious cycle of gaining and losing weight. Not only have they kept their weight down for years, but they have improved their posture, strengthened their bones, achieved a greater level of self-esteem, and vastly enhanced their overall health.

Don't Be Afraid of Muscles

I know my female readers are saying to themselves, "I don't want big muscles. I just want to be toned." Trust me, you are not going to develop bulging biceps, but you will appear, to use the popular expression, "toned." After the age of twenty, the average individual (men as well as women) loses one-half to seven-tenths of a pound of muscle each year. That's right, you are losing muscle each and every day. And, as you will read in Chapter 9, as a woman nears menopause, she begins to lose muscle at almost *twice* that rate. Therefore, even to maintain your existing muscle, you need to perform strength and resistance exercise on a regular basis. Nothing else gets the job done.

Women shouldn't fear muscle or worry that strength and resistance exercise will turn them into muscle-bound clones of the females depicted in bodybuilder magazines. The women in those magazines, like their male counterparts, are following an extreme eating and exercise regimen that usually includes the use of some type of food supplement or steroid.

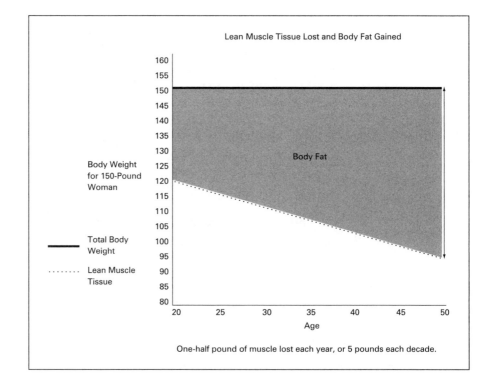

Lean Muscle Tissue Lost and Body Fat Gained

Body Weight for 150-Pound Woman

Body Fat

Total Body Weight

Lean Muscle Tissue

One-half pound of muscle lost each year, or 5 pounds each decade.

The Visual

Take a look at the opposite graphics, which represent cross sections of women's thighs, adapted from *Strong Women Stay Young* by Miriam Nelson, who holds a doctorate in nutrition and is also a sports medicine specialist at Tufts University, and Sarah Wernick.

Clearly, the moderately active young woman and the older woman who strength trains have almost identical thighs. This is such a great visual regarding what is happening on the inside when you perform strength and resistance exercise. Which graphic do you think represents you?

So, You Want to Look "Toned"

Let's examine what so many women refer to as "toning." A so-called toned visual occurs when body fat is burned off of an area of the body and the muscle underneath is maintained, or slightly increased in size. This produces the toned effect. Strength and resistance exercise creates this visual by building the muscle underneath and simultaneously boosting your metabolism, which enables you to burn body fat to reveal the muscle. You essentially receive two benefits for the price of one type of exercise and create the "toned" body you desire. Keep in mind, the strength and resistance exercise *always* should be complemented with a low-calorie eating plan if weight loss is your goal.

Listen to This Jane

In the *Wall Street Journal,* Jane Brody, who writes a frequent column on personal health, puts it very simply; she says, "Strength training leads to a smaller, tighter physique." I couldn't agree more.

I know this may sound confusing. We have been brainwashed for so long by weight-loss books, arti-

STRENGTH TRAINING BUILDS MUSCLE

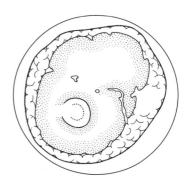

Moderately Active Young Woman

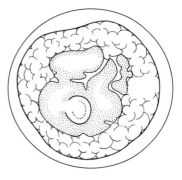

Sedentary Middle-Age Woman
She has less muscle and more fat than the younger woman, primarily because she is inactive, not becasue of her age.

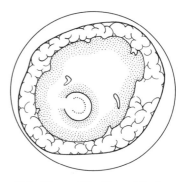

Older Woman Who Strength Trains
Her thigh is similar to the thigh of the younger woman.

cles, or celebrity-endorsed programs that constantly promote cardiovascular exercise as the key to weight loss. Did they work? No. The models used in the promos look good. Will the models continue to look good without embracing strength and resistance exercise? No. Stop and think about this point. During the time that the exercise explosion occurred in this country, the average American grew in size—considerably.

Don't Listen to This Jane

The United States became enamored with exercise programs in the 1970s—aerobics of all types, Jane Fonda, high-impact aerobics, low-impact aerobics, you name it. I wanted to lose weight so I joined right in. At the time this emphasis on cardiovascular exercise was taking place, what was occurring throughout the United States? Weight gain. Men, women, teenagers, and children gained huge amounts of weight. How ironic. We as a nation became obsessed with exercise at the same time the weight-gain epidemic took hold throughout the country. In my mind this is a strong piece of evidence indicating that cardiovascular exercise isn't the correct form of exercise to achieve successful weight loss. We need a new approach and that needs to be strength and resistance exercise.

Put Cardio in Proper Perspective
A Little Bit Goes a Long Way

I'm not saying that one should never do cardiovascular exercise. Cardiovascular exercise challenges the body's most important muscle, the heart. My program encourages you to perform brief periods of cardiovascular exercise, with a maximum of fifteen minutes. (You'll find detailed guidelines on the role of cardiovascular exercise in my workouts starting on page 190 of this chapter.) But, except for those preparing for the Olympics, professional athletes, or those who wish to participate in marathons, prolonged periods of cardiovascular exercise are absolutely *not* the key to weight loss. Once again, the human body is very smart. When you first begin performing a cardiovascular activity, whether it's walking, running, stepping, spinning, stair climbing, etc., you do burn additional calories. But as your body becomes more capable of performing that activity, the amount of energy, or calories expended, diminishes.

It is exactly like the cruise-control option on your car. Why do you use it? To conserve energy, or gas, by keeping your car's speed at a consistent rate. Do you want to conserve energy when you exercise? Absolutely not. Consequently, to continue to burn additional calories, you have to keep running farther, or faster, or uphill, or whatever to keep burning the *same* number of calories. Your body is being abused because you are in a vicious cycle of pushing it harder, harder, and harder. If you continue, the likelihood of an injury occurring is high, which will terminate your exercise program. This definitely is not what I want for you. I want you to adopt an exercise regimen that is a proven formula for successful, permanent weight loss. That formula is based upon strength and resistance exercise.

DON'T FLIP THE CRUISE CONTROL ON

Exercise for Life

My goal is for you to be able to exercise for the rest of your life. Honestly, you should plan on performing strength and resistance exercise forever. When you read Chapter 10, "'It's Just Too Late,'" you will understand its importance, especially as you age; it becomes a necessity to maintain the quality of your life. The elderly have more to gain than anyone when it comes to the benefits of strength and resistance exercise. It can almost solely determine the quality of their life in their latter years.

And younger readers should realize that what I am telling you today will be considered the norm in the future. You, too, are going to become a senior citizen and what will get you to and through those "golden" years is a well-thought-out weight-management program that incorporates strength and resistance exercise.

"Tip" the Flip

A year or so ago, a client recommended *The Tipping Point* by Malcolm Gladwell. I found it extremely thought-provoking. Gladwell describes how trends or changes occur in our society, whether it's fashion, television programming, even crime rates. According to Gladwell, these changes occur when the "word" gets out and thus a new style, philosophy, or belief starts to "tip." My goal is to "tip" the scales toward the flip. I want Americans to reach *the tipping point* to *flip the switch* and realize that the key to weight loss is strength and resistance, not cardiovascular, exercise. I believe, just as I urged you to believe in your ability to lose weight, that I will be successful in this endeavor. So, you can hang on to your treadmill; just don't plan on spending any more than a few minutes on it if you want to achieve weight loss.

To put these changing times and facts into perspective, consider the following statements that were once widely regarded as fact:

What We Once Thought Was True

- The earth is flat.

- The earth is the center of the solar system.

- Women are inferior to men.

- Chocolate causes acne.

- Man will never land on the moon.

- You can eat all you want and lose weight.

- The "Wonder Weighted Belt" is the key to reducing your midsection.

- Cardiovascular exercise is the secret to weight loss.

Times change, knowledge and information change, and we all need to incorporate new information into our lives. That's what learning is all about.

Why Are Health Club Memberships *and* Waistlines Increasing? An American Paradox

Today, both the number of obese Americans and the number of health club memberships is on the rise. According to the International Health, Racquet, and Sportsclub Association, "Memberships grew from 21 million in 1991 to 30.6 million in 1999." If health club memberships are on the rise and the number of overweight Americans is on the rise, what's going on? My take is that, yes, *some* people are

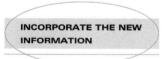

INCORPORATE THE NEW
INFORMATION

joining and *some* are working out in those clubs. Unfortunately, most likely they are performing the wrong style of exercise or taking gimmicky classes such as karaoke spinning. Most are attending aerobics class or using the treadmill, bike, stair climber, elliptical trainer, and rower. All should be in the strength and resistance exercise room. That produces weight loss.

They Kept Running, They Kept Gaining

Here's one last bit of information that may convert you to my camp. The Lawrence Berkeley National Laboratory in Berkeley, California, surveyed runners and found that those who continued to run the same distance from age twenty to fifty gained on average 3.3 pounds and three-quarters of an inch at the waist each decade. Think about that. These people kept running the same distance and gained weight and inches! What was happening? They were losing muscle as they aged and the cardiovascular exercise chewed it up even more. Only strength and resistance exercise can consistently enable you to lose weight and inches. Furthermore, this survey didn't take into consideration the fact that most individuals cannot continue to run the same mileage each year for thirty years. Odds are, an injury will derail this exercise program well before thirty years elapse.

Gayle Did It

As I am finishing this book, I am working on a project with *O, The Oprah Magazine.* Four women have agreed to go on the Jim Karas plan for weight loss. One of my four participants is Gayle King, editor-at-large of *O, The Oprah Magazine,* and Oprah's best friend. Gayle is in her late forties and was a religious cardiovascular exerciser. Like so many others, she said to me when we first met, "I thought cardio was the

TAKE ANOTHER JIM KARAS CHALLENGE

Go to your nearest health club or gym and observe the people in the cardiovascular room and then the strength and resistance room. Which group appears more fit? Draw your own conclusion.

ARE YOU RUNNING TO LOSE OR RUNNING TO GAIN?

IT TAKES LESS TIME THAN YOU THINK

I bet you think you have to perform hour after hour of strength and exercise training to see benefits. You must think it will take forever. Guess what? Dr. Miriam Nelson states that "in just four weeks of two 40-minute sessions a week, you will see a distinct improvement in your strength and well-being." Four weeks and a total of eighty minutes a week, and for years we were led to believe we had to exercise for hours and hours on end. Wrong!

key to weight loss." Gayle definitely falls into the Slow-Gainer pattern of weight gain. She just added a few pounds here, a few pounds there, and ultimately started my program at 174.6 pounds. (Gayle has a scale that gives her weight in tenths, and she always tells me the exact number.) She was very clear about one point: "I don't want to start a program of eating and exercise that I can't stick with," she said. "I'm not going to do one of those extreme programs." I totally agreed with her. I said, "Let's try counting your calories, eating around sixteen hundred calories a day and embracing my style of exercise, strength and resistance training." She agreed.

In three months, Gayle is down approximately twenty pounds. By six months, almost twenty-five pounds. She is back in her size 10 clothes, which she really likes, and even they are starting to get big. Her arms have changed. The whole composition of her body has changed. By the time you read this book, I'm positive she will have lost even more weight and inches. Like Diane Sawyer, she is inspiring so many women (including many at *O* and at the Oxygen Network, where she hosts a talk show) to embrace strength and resistance exercise. Why? Because it works. They see the change. They ask me, "Can I do the same?" I always ask, "Are you currently performing strength and resistance exercise?" Ninety-nine times out of one hundred the answer is the same: "No, I do cardio." They won't get results like Gayle's unless they change their approach to exercise.

Are You Hungry?

I have one final point to make on cardiovascular exercise: Mind you, I started my own exercise program more than twenty years ago as a runner. Do you know what I found? I found that I was starving all the time and eating more than I should have been. Here I was, running, only to be eating even more calories because I was so damn hungry. My Balance of Energy Equation was:

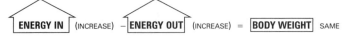

ENERGY IN (INCREASE) − ENERGY OUT (INCREASE) = BODY WEIGHT SAME

I heard Joy Behar, one of the hosts of ABC's *The View,* say that all cardiovascular exercise does is make her hungry. She's right. Does this

THIS IS A PROGRAM
YOU CAN DO FOR LIFE

WHAT'S
KEPT *YOU*
FROM
FLIPPING?

178

apply to you? Are you eating extra calories because you are performing all this cardiovascular exercise?

How Are You Feeling?

Before I give you your strength and resistance exercise plans, I want to explore your past and present relationship to exercise just as I did with your relationship to food. As we have done so often in this journey to flipping, I want to know how you feel about your physical ability. To do so, I want you to complete the sentence: *When I was young, physically I felt . . .* (Use the space provided at right.)

My response would be the following: *When I was young, physically I felt weak. I had asthma, so I couldn't run without the fear of an attack. I couldn't catch a ball. No one ever taught me how and I was afraid of the ball. I didn't play sports because I observed the coaches always yelling at the players and I didn't want to get yelled at. There was enough yelling in my home growing up. I didn't need any more. I was always picked last for teams in gym class, because, quite frankly, I wouldn't have wanted me on the team either. Basically I was fat, afraid, and bad at each and every sport.*

Writing that was not fun. When I stop and reread what I just wrote, it's quite painful, but it's the truth. I realize that I missed out on a lot, not only the physical benefits that the exercise would have provided but the social aspects as well. It was not until my early twenties that I started exercising and began to change my relationship to exercise. Thus, our second exercise—complete the sentence: *Now, physically I feel . . .* (Use the space provided on page 180.)

Here is my response: *Now, physically I feel the strongest I have felt in my life. I enjoy playing sports. I have no injuries because I have taken care of my body by*

EXERCISE 1

"I HATE TO EXERCISE"

When I was young, physically I felt . . .

"I HATE TO EXERCISE"

Now, physically I feel . . .

_____

_____

_____

_____

_____

_____

_____

_____

_____

_____

_____

_____

_____

_____

_____

strengthening it. It never, never crosses my mind that I may not be able to physically do something. I am actually very proud that at forty-one, I feel I am in the same shape as someone decades younger.

And: *At my recent twenty-year high school reunion, many of the former athletes, even the so-called star athletes who never wanted me on their teams, had gained a tremendous amount of weight. Irony of ironies, I, the nonjock fatty, was now the strong, lean one; I have to admit it made me smile, just a little, inside. If I can do it, so can you.*

Mind you, this change didn't happen overnight. It took time. Remember, I started my exercise program by running. Yes, yes, we're back to cardiovascular exercise, because that was what we were led to believe in the early 1980s was the key to weight loss. Everyone was doing it. After doing this for a while (and suffering terrible shin splints), I started going to a gym and performing strength and resistance exercise. Within a month, I noticed that I was beginning to lose weight and my body's composition was changing. I actually started to have a waist! I always use myself as a case study when I research exercise programs, and I found that the strength and resistance exercise was the "magic pill" when it comes to losing weight. Plus, I just loved seeing the results (my first experience with a *positive* visualization of my body) of all my hard work when I looked in the mirror.

Getting Started

For many of us, the first attempt at exercise can make a significant difference. We all know how important a first impression can be. That's why I am going to present you with three exercise programs, which you'll find beginning on page 189 of this chapter, all fully illustrated for easy reference. The first two of these programs can be performed in your home or office; only the third program necessitates going to a gym or health club. I purposely designed the exercise programs this way because I want *you* to determine which exercise environment is best for you. In Chapter 3, "'I Don't Have the Time,'" you determined the time of day that's best for you to exercise. Now decide if you feel more comfortable in the privacy of your home or office. It's possible that you may like the equipment, energy, and social aspect of a gym or health club. The choice is yours. Base the choice on what will best lead you to success. Don't allow someone to influence your decision. You know yourself better than others do. The goal is for *you* to be a success at weight loss, not necessarily a success at pleasing others.

The Comfort Room

I frequently hear women, and occasionally a few men, state that in their gym or health club they do only cardiovascular exercise because it is the room where they feel "most comfortable." Many have said that they once or twice ventured into the strength and resistance exercise rooms, but they didn't know what they were doing and consequently felt out of place. They further stated that if they did attempt to use the strength and resistance exercise equipment, they ended up plopping down on the first piece of equipment they came upon, not knowing how to adjust the seat, the pads, or the weight, and struggled to perform the exercise.

One woman (my editor, Becky Cabaza) told me that she caught a glimpse of herself in the mirror as she tried to work one machine and realized that her feet were not touching the floor. She felt like a little kid in a grown-up's chair, feet dangling away. Obviously the machine setting was incorrect for her size. Becky said that when she first began using the machines, she was too intimidated to ask for help. I realize this can frequently happen. That's why you may opt to begin your exercise program in your home or at your office. This way you can perfect your strength and resistance exercise technique and then acquire the confidence to overcome the intimidating aspect of a gym or health club. Trust me, your confidence will quickly grow. (And remember, you're paying for that membership, so ask for some service and get a trainer to show you how to use the equipment!)

IT'S TIME TO EXPLORE THE *OTHER* PART OF THE GYM

One Woman's Victory: Yesssss!

I recently read an article by a woman who had experienced the benefits of strength and resistance exercise. Guess what really jumped off the page as I was reading? The day finally came at the gym when she was waiting for a man to finish his set on the leg-press machine. After he was done, he looked her over and started to pull off the forty-five-pound plates, assuming she would be doing less weight. She said to him, "No, no, don't do that. Keep them on and if you could, please add another ten pounds to each side." Inside she said to herself, "Yesssss!" I love that story. She obviously experienced a great feeling of accomplishment. You, too, can feel the same.

Prepare Yourself for "The Room"

Think about this point. I don't want you to go to a club, change your clothes, grab your water bottle and this book, and venture into the strength and resistance exercise room or the "free weight" room, which is often separate from the area where the strength and resistance machines are located, only to be put off by the other people in the room.

Keep in mind, everyone in that room was once a novice and didn't know what to do. Many still don't. Countless number of men—yes, men—are in these rooms performing exercises incorrectly. Most of the men probably had their buddies take them through their first routine.

Advance Planning and Time Management

Once again, you can successfully maneuver this environment by employing advance planning and the time-management elements we discussed earlier. Clearly, at prime time, in the early morning or right after work, the strength and resistance exercise room at a health club or gym will be more crowded. To deal with this, it might be best for you to start on a weekend, in the middle of the day, or at some time that you know would afford you more access to the equipment without someone breathing down your neck and watching you. Do some research. Ask the floor person or other club management when it is less crowded. However, if you are ready to do

EVERYONE WAS A
NOVICE ONCE

this at prime time, go for it. Does it really matter what your fellow exercisers think? Of course not. Most of them are too absorbed in their own routines or appearances to closely focus on anyone but themselves. Just say to yourself, "If they can do it, so can I. I will be a success in this room."

The Rules

Here are a few guidelines you need to follow when performing any of the three strength and resistance exercise plans:

1. The speed in which you perform strength and resistance exercises is critically important. I want you to begin by always counting slowly to three as you pull or press the weight machine, the SPRI tubing, or the dumbbells, hold for one count (unless otherwise specified) at the end of each repetition, then release for a slow three count back to the starting position. For the record, the counting is *one one thousand, two one thousand, three one thousand, hold one thousand. . . .* Slow repetitions are the key to an effective, injury-free workout.

2. Perform one set of each exercise, to start. Each "set" should consist of no more than eight to ten repetitions, or "reps," of each exercise. If an exercise requires you to work first one side of your body, then the other, you should perform eight to ten repetitions

EASE IN AT "OFF PEAK"

When I first began to visit a gym, I went into the weight room at off-peak times since I felt I needed extra time to understand the equipment and was intimidated. But after a handful of visits, I had the confidence to go at any time and felt great. You may want to try the same off-peak approach, if you're having trouble getting started.

COUNT SLOWLY

THINK STRONG TO
GET STRONG

on each side. Eventually, you may work up to twelve reps. (You'll read more about the function of reps later in this chapter.)

3. Focus your mind on the muscles you are working. Researchers have noted that just *thinking* about strengthening your muscles can help strengthen them. Dr. Finoth Ranganathan, with a team of researchers from the Cleveland Clinic in Ohio, split thirty healthy young adults into three groups. One group imagined exercising their little finger, one group their biceps, and one group served as a control group who performed no visualization exercise. After twelve weeks of performing this for fifteen minutes five days a week, the finger exercisers increased their strength by 35 percent and the biceps group increased theirs by 13.4 percent. The control group had no change. Think back for a moment on Chapter 2 and my discussion of the power of mind-body visualization. The mind actually has the power to make your muscles stronger. Couple this realization with the strength and resistance exercises I will soon prescribe and you have the perfect blend of the mind and body working in tandem to achieve one goal—an increase in lean muscle tissue and a boost in your metabolism that leads to weight loss.

4. Drink water. It is important that you grasp how essential water is to your success. When you perform strength and resistance exercise, you are asking your muscles to expand and contract. Remember, muscles are composed of 60 to 70 percent water. Therefore, you will derive more benefit from the workout if you are well hydrated. A small tip for those of you who will be exercising first thing in the morning: The water you consume the night before will make a huge difference when you work out in the morning as will minimizing or eliminating your alcohol, sodium, and caffeine intake. So drink lots of water the night before, be careful with sodium, alcohol, and caffeine, and always, always drink plenty of water before, during, and after each exercise session.

5. Breathe. I know this direction sounds obvious, but many individuals hold their breath during strength and resistance exercises. As a general rule, you should exhale on the exertion, or the hard part, and inhale as you release. Also, breathe through both your nose and mouth if possible. That way, you will take in more oxygen with each breath. I recommend that you inhale slowly, as if you have a straw in your mouth. Exhale the same way.

6. Tuck your abdominals. I am repeatedly going to instruct you to keep your abdominals tucked during each exercise. By tucking, I mean you should pull your abs in to provide support for your abdominal and lower back area. Right now, just place your hand on your stomach and pull it in. You will visually see and feel your muscles pull in. That is the position I want you to assume when I say "tuck." Fitness professionals call this area the "core" as it is the foundation of your body. In doing so, you will functionally strengthen your body and support it as you trim your waist and abdominal area. By doing this, you will derive two benefits for the price of one exercise. You'll notice that I recommend only one abdominal exercise per session (that is really all you need), but I expect you to keep your abdominals tucked while performing *all* of the exercises in your program, not just the abdominal exercises.

DON'T HOLD YOUR
BREATH, AND KEEP
YOUR ABS TUCKED

The Exercise Prescription:
25 Percent Cardiovascular,
75 Percent Strength and Resistance

So that we are clear, that means that if you plan to exercise for twenty minutes, you would perform cardiovascular exercise for five minutes.

DON'T I HAVE TO DO SOME CARDIOVASCULAR EXERCISE?

Yes. While I have repeatedly told you that exclusive cardiovascular exercise is not the key to weight loss, it is necessary for you to perform cardio for a few minutes before each strength and resistance exercise workout (read about the benefits of cardiovascular exercise at right). Here is the percentage: I want you to spend 25 percent of the time you have to exercise on cardio and the remaining 75 percent on strength and resistance training.

If you plan to exercise for forty minutes, then you would perform cardio for ten minutes, and so on. Cardiovascular exercise produces the following benefits:

- *It warms up your body for strength and resistance exercise.* Your body's "core" temperature needs to rise prior to applying resistance. That rise occurs during cardiovascular exercise. Therefore, your cardio time doubles as an opportunity for your body to prepare for the strength and resistance exercise. Look at cardio as your "warm-up act" and the strength and resistance exercise as the "headliner."

- *It works the most important muscle of the body—the heart.* Cardiovascular exercise challenges the heart. Strength and resistance training challenges the heart as well, but the intensity when exclusively performing cardiovascular exercise is generally slightly higher. More on intensity below.

- *It helps beat the blues.* Cardiovascular exercise produces a number of benefits when it comes to depression and anxiety, as does strength and resistance training. The cardio will jump-start this process and then the strength and resistance exercise will carry it through.

The key to cardiovascular exercise is the intensity. Strolling will generally produce little if no result, unless you are so terribly out of shape that your heart is pounding. I constantly observe people taking a leisurely walk on treadmills. Unless they plan on performing this exercise for hours and hours on end, they will burn few if any calories. Remember, we are in the calorie-burning business. That is why you are going to perform strength and resistance exercise, which burns calories twenty-four hours a day, seven days a week.

Listen to Your Body, Especially Your Heart

Take your heart rate, which, if you remember, I taught you to do in Chapter 4. See where the exercise is taking your body in terms of beats per minute. You might consider investing in a heart-rate monitor. Take a look at the options available at my website, www.jimkaras.com and click on exercise equipment.

Once you are comfortable, don't be afraid of pushing. On the contrary, all the the benefits mentioned are enhanced when you challenge your body. Your heart will thank you, you'll warm up faster, and your emotional well-being will vastly improve.

How Fast Should Your Heart Beat During Cardiovascular Exercise?

That depends on a number of factors. They include your current fitness level, any medications you take, the climate you are exercising in, and your age. The older you are, the lower you should aim to keep your heart rate.

Here are some parameters:

AGE	OPTIMAL BEATS PER MINUTE
20	154–187
25	150–182
30	147–178
35	143–174
40	140–170
45	136–165
50	133–161
55	129–157

GET INTO THE CALORIE-BURNING BUSINESS

Please get a complete physical or consult your primary-care physician before starting this or any exercise program, especially if you are on medication or have any specific health concerns.

AGE	OPTIMAL BEATS PER MINUTE
60	126–153
65	122–148
70	119–144
75	115–140
80	112–136

I'll Have a Little Cardio with My Strength Training

Here are just a few ideas for your cardiovascular warm-up:

- Walking or running outside, inside, or on a treadmill. If you run, just be careful with your joints and make sure to wear a good, new pair of running shoes. If you can find a soft outdoor track to run on, great. Same goes for the treadmill, which generally is softer on your joints.

- Stepping on the bottom step of a staircase or with one of the step products on the market. Just stepping up and down, up and down, rapidly gets your heart rate up. You may also climb full flights of stairs. Just be careful on the way down as you could hurt your knees. While it's more challenging to climb stairs than to descend them, you put a tremendous amount of pressure on your knees going down.

- Cycling inside or outside. Hop on your bike or use a stationary bicycle in your home or office. It is generally better for your knees as it does not require impact on the joints.

- Skipping or jumping rope. Jumping rope is very intense. Be careful with your joints and jump in the proper shoes and on as soft a surface as possible. It can be done anywhere and it's cheap.

- Gym or health club equipment. Cardiovascular pieces of equipment in a club include the elliptical trainer, the rower (I only really like the Concept II, which truly replicates the rowing movement), the Versa Climber (which is extremely difficult—ask for help from a trainer), one of the stair-climbing machines, or the ergometer (which uses your arms rather than your lower body—a good choice for those with injuries to the lower body that prohibit them from impact on the legs or spine). All of these are just fine. Give them a try.

The Workouts: Three Ways to Flip

For those of you who have been dreading physical exercise, the time is now. Don't be frightened. Unlike your past attempts, this time it's different. You're prepared: You've read this book; you've flipped; you've done the essential mental homework. You firmly believe you can be a success. You visualized your success. You found the time, the energy, and the money to flip. You cast aside the belief that your present weight was the fault of your genes or metabolism. You are learning to eat in a more calorie-controlled manner and now, finally, you are ready to tackle another essential component to a successful flip: strength and resistance exercise.

WHAT ABOUT SWIMMING?

Swimming may not be your best choice because you have to get out, dry off, change, and then perform your strength and resistance exercise. While I sometimes swim on vacation for ten to fifteen minutes, that is generally in the middle of the day after I have performed my strength and resistance exercise. Research indicates that swimming leads to a higher percentage of body fat, as the body holds additional fat to stay afloat and keep warm in the generally cool water. But if swimming is your favorite form of cardio, then by all means get wet, get your heart rate up, and burn some calories, which intense swimming will do.

FLIP
THE SWITCH

STRENGTH
AND
RESISTANCE
EXERCISE

Flip the Switch Strength and Resistance Training Program 1 with SPRI* Xertube, Xering, and Resist-A-Ball

*See page 100 for information on purchasing SPRI products.

⇨ Staying on the Ball

If you're feeling a bit unsure about being able to perform certain exercises atop the Resist-A-Ball, rest assured that it's much easier than it looks. Still, if you're concerned about being able to keep your balance, simply position yourself near a wall, chair, table, or other support. You may also choose not to inflate the ball all the way. When you sit on a ball that has not been inflated to capacity, your body weight will naturally cause you to "sink" into the ball; the area of the ball that makes contact with the floor will be larger, so it will not roll as easily. After a few workouts, you will feel very confident about using this effective and ingenious piece of equipment. My clients love it.

⇨ Attaching the Xertube

The exercises in Program 1 instruct you to place the door attachment for the Xertube "next to" the doorknob, though in many photos you'll see that the attachment is well above or below the doorknob. The exact placement of the attachment depends on the height of the doorknob and on your height as well. Refer to the door attachment instructions for more information, and take your height and the position of the doorknob into account.

⇨ Muscle in on these terms

ABS—Abdominal muscles, located in your abdomen

PECS—Pectoral muscles, located in your chest

BICEPS—Located in the front of your arm

TRICEPS—Located in the back of your arm

DELTS—Deltoid muscles, located in your shoulders

GLUTES—Gluteus maximus muscles, located in your rear end (yes, there are muscles in there)

HAMSTRINGS—located along the back of your thigh

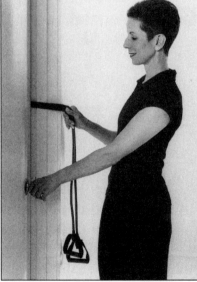

Attach the xertube to the door, adjusting the height to each exercise

TEN EXERCISES WITH SPRI XERTUBE, XERING, AND RESIST-A-BALL

Perform 8 to 10 repetitions of each exercise.

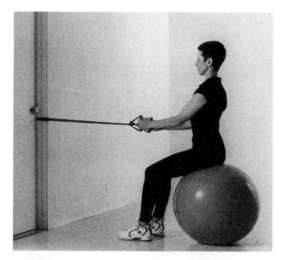

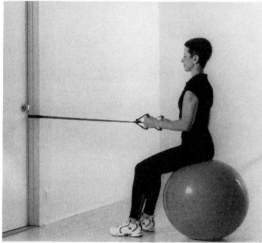

1. Seated Back Row on Ball

1. Place the Xertube in the door attachment and attach it next to the doorknob.

2. Place the Resist-A-Ball approximately four feet from the door.

3. Sit on the ball with your feet shoulder-width apart, toes forward, and abdominals tucked.

4. Grasp the Xertube with your palms facing each other and pull your shoulders back.

5. Slowly exhale as you pull the Xertube toward you and hold.

6. Concentrate on pulling your shoulder blades together.

7. Slowly inhale as you release.

8. Make sure to sit upright at all times and try not to lean back.

"I HATE TO EXERCISE"

191

2. Rear Deltoid Fly on Ball

1. Place the Xertube in the door attachment and attach it next to the doorknob.

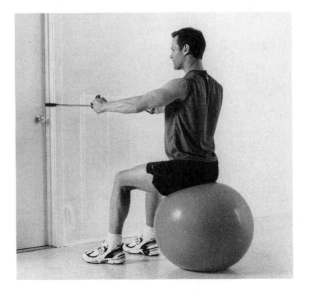

2. Place the Resist-A-Ball approximately three feet from the door. If that is too difficult, move closer.

3. Sit on the ball with your feet shoulder-width apart, toes forward, and abdominals tucked.

4. Grasp the Xertube with your palms facing each other and pull your shoulders back.

5. Slowly exhale as you pull the Xertube out and then back with slightly bent arms. (Note: This is a fly movement, not a row as in the first exercise.)

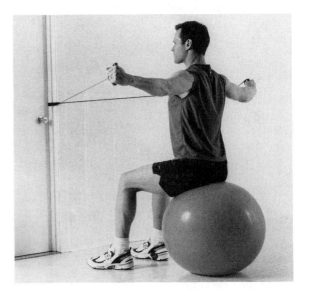

6. Hold for one count, then slowly inhale as you return.

7. Make sure to sit upright at all times and try not to lean back.

3. Chest Press on Ball

1. Place the Xertube in the door attachment and attach it next to the doorknob.

2. Place the Resist-A-Ball approximately two feet from the door.

3. Sit on the ball facing away from the door (the opposite of the first two exercises) with your feet shoulder-width apart, toes pointed forward, and abdominals tucked.

4. Grasp the Xertube with your palms facing forward and your elbows on the same plane as your shoulders.

5. Slowly exhale as you press the Xertube out as you squeeze your pecs (chest muscles).

6. Hold for one count, then inhale as you release until your elbows are on the same plane as your shoulders.

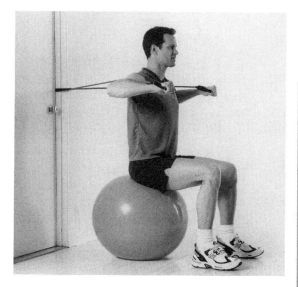

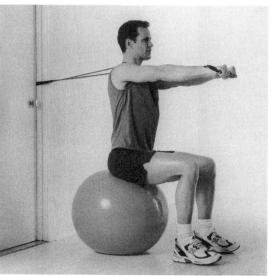

4. Standing Biceps Curl

1. Stand with your feet shoulder-width apart, toes forward, and abdominals tucked.

2. Place the Xertube under both feet and grasp the handles with your palms facing up.

3. Slowly exhale as you curl your arms up, hold, then inhale as you release.

4. Concentrate on your biceps and squeeze them as you curl the Xertube up.

5. Make sure to keep your shoulders and neck relaxed at all times.

6. Keep your wrists strong. Don't let them bend back.

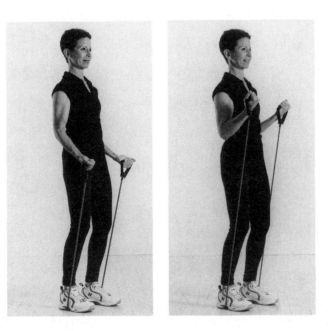

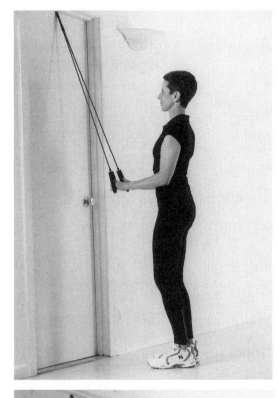

5. Triceps Pushdown

1. Place the Xertube in the door attachment and secure at the top of the door.

2. Stand with your feet shoulder-width apart, toes forward, and abdominals tucked.

3. Grasp the Xertube with your palms facing down with your elbows secure at your sides.

4. Slowly exhale as you press your arms down and hold; inhale as you release.

5. Concentrate on your triceps and squeeze them as you press the Xertube down.

6. Make sure to keep your shoulders and neck relaxed at all times.

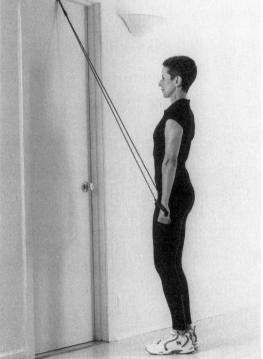

6. Hip Extension

1. Place the Xering around both feet.

2. Place your arms at your sides, on your hips or use a chair or wall for balance. Abdominals tucked.

3. Shift your weight to your right leg; lift the left slightly off of the floor.

4. Slowly exhale as you press the left leg back and hold.

5. Inhale as you return and keep the left leg off of the floor until all repetitions are completed.

6. Concentrate on your glutes (the muscles in your rear end) throughout the exercise.

7. You will feel this exercise in both your left and right glutes.

8. Repeat on the right leg.

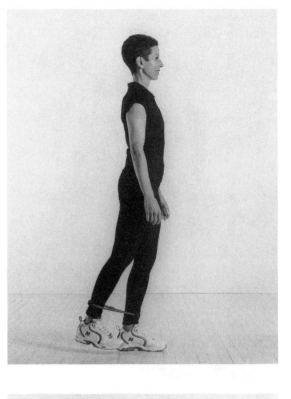

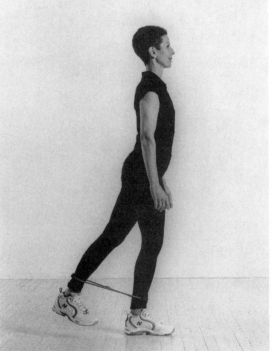

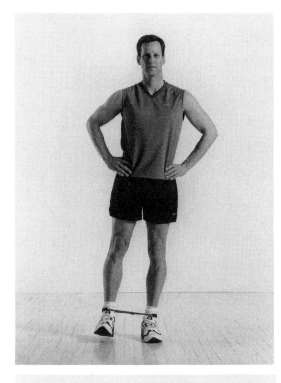

7. Hip Abduction

1. Place the Xering around both feet.

2. Place your arms at your sides, on your hips or use a chair or wall for balance. Abdominals tucked.

3. Shift your weight to your left leg; lift the right slightly off of the floor.

4. Slowly exhale as you press the right leg out to your side and hold.

5. Inhale as you return and keep the right leg off of the floor until all repetitions are completed.

6. Concentrate on your glutes (the muscles in your rear end) and hips throughout the exercise.

7. You will feel this exercise in both your left and right glutes and each hip (the right hip when you lift the right leg, then the left hip when you lift the left leg).

8. Repeat on the left leg.

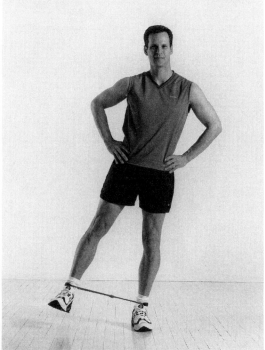

8. Side Steps with Xering

1. Place the Xering around both feet.

2. Place your arms at your sides or on your hips and assume a quarter squat position, abdominals tucked.

3. Start with your feet together, then step out with the right leg.

4. Slowly let the left leg come halfway back toward your right while resisting the tension.

5. Repeat going the other way.

6. At all times, maintain a degree of tension and stay in the partial squat.

7. You should feel the exercise in both glutes and both hips.

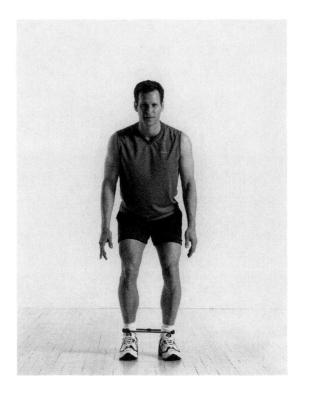

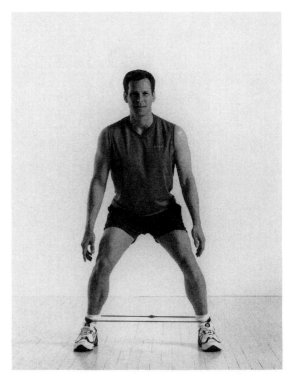

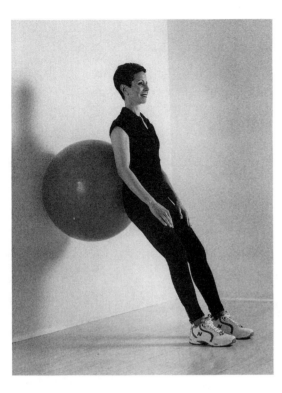

9. Ball Wall Squats

1. Place the Resist-A-Ball against a secure wall.

2. Position the ball in the small of your back.

3. Place your feet shoulder-width apart with toes forward, abdominals tucked.

4. Slowly inhale as you lower yourself down until your hamstrings (the muscles in back of your thighs) are parallel to the floor.

5. Exhale as you squeeze your glutes and press up through your heels.

6. Lift up until your knees are slightly bent— in other words, don't lock them.

7. Keep your shoulders back and your chin in alignment at all times.

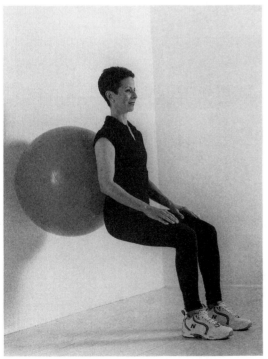

10. Abs with Xertube

1. Place the Xertube in the door attachment and attach it above the doorknob.

2. Place the Resist-A-Ball approximately three feet from the door.

3. Sit on the ball with your feet shoulder-width apart, toes forward, and abdominals tucked.

4. As pictured, sit facing at a 90-degree angle from the door.

5. Grasp both handles in your left hand and fold your right hand over.

6. With extended arms, slowly twist away from the door and hold.

7. Your eyes should follow your hands at all times.

8. Concentrate on your abdominals at all times; don't just "muscle through" with your arms.

9. Repeat on the other side.

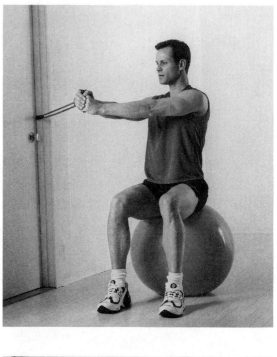

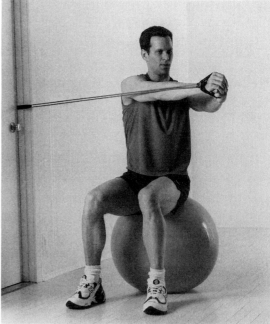

TEN EXERCISES WITH FREE WEIGHTS* AND RESIST-A-BALL

*See page 223 for information on how much weight to use.

Perform 8 to 10 repetitions of each exercise.

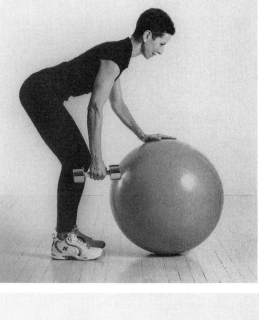

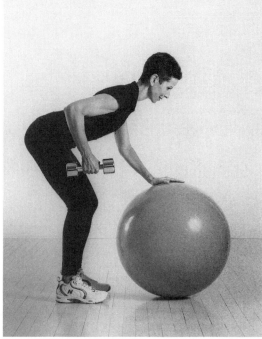

1. One-Arm Row with Ball

1. Place your feet shoulder-width apart with toes forward.

2. Grasp your dumbbell in your right hand; place your left hand on the ball.

3. Slowly roll the ball forward as you lean over until your back is flat.

4. Keep your head and chin in alignment as pictured.

5. As you exhale, slowly pull the dumbbell up until it almost touches your chest.

6. Inhale as you release, but keep a slight bend in your elbow at the bottom.

7. At all times, tuck your abdominals to support your lower back.

8. Make sure that you do not lift your working shoulder, only the arm.

9. Repeat on the other side.

"I HATE TO EXERCISE"

201

2. Chest Press with Ball

1. Sit on the Resist-A-Ball with your toes facing forward, feet shoulder-width apart, and grasp one dumbbell in each hand.

2. Slowly walk your feet forward until your head and upper shoulders are supported by the ball.

3. Tuck your abdominals and lift your lower back so that your body is parallel to the floor—this is starting position.

4. With your palms facing forward, slowly exhale as you press the dumbbells up; inhale as you release back to starting position.

5. Squeeze your chest as you lift but do not lock your elbows at the top; keep them slightly bent.

6. Make sure that your abdominals and lower back remain in starting position—don't let your body sink as you proceed through the set.

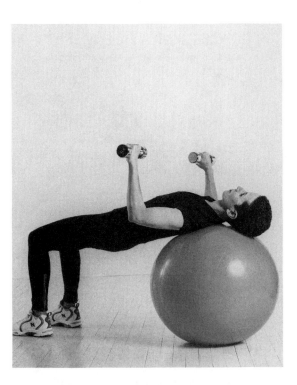

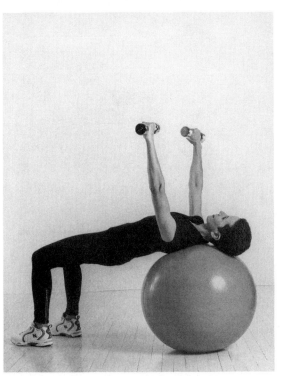

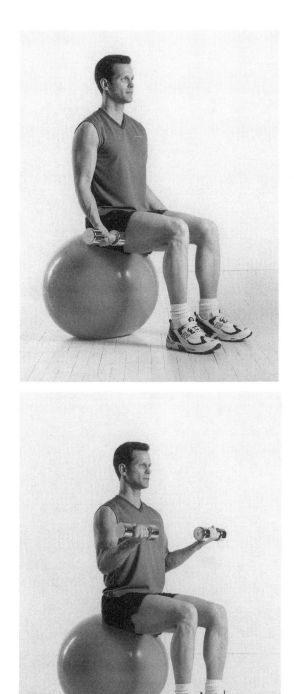

3. Bicep Curl with Ball

1. Sit on the Resist-A-Ball with your feet shoulder-width apart and toes forward.

2. Grasp one dumbbell in each hand with your elbows tucked at your sides.

3. Sit straight up with your shoulders back and abdominals tucked.

4. Slowly exhale as you curl the dumbbells up with your palms facing up; slowly inhale as you release to starting position to where the elbow is slightly bent.

5. The curl is finished when your elbow starts to move up from your side.

6. Make sure to keep your shoulders and neck relaxed at all times.

7. Keep your wrists strong. Don't let them bend back.

4. Tricep Extension

1. Lie on your back on the floor with your feet firmly planted on the floor, shoulder-width apart.

2. Grasp one dumbbell in each hand and extend your arms over your head.

3. Your palms face each other at all times and your wrists stay in alignment.

4. Slowly inhale as you lower the dumbbells alongside your ears, then exhale as you press your arms back up to starting position.

5. Keep your abdominals tucked at all times to support your lower back.

6. Make sure to keep your shoulders and neck relaxed at all times.

Training tip:

If you feel pressure in your neck, you might want to roll a small towel under your neck for support.

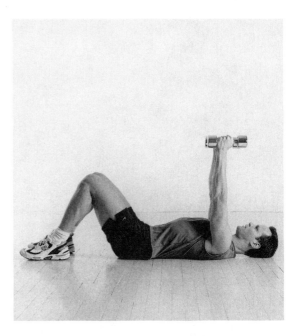

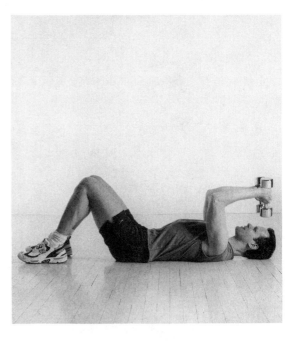

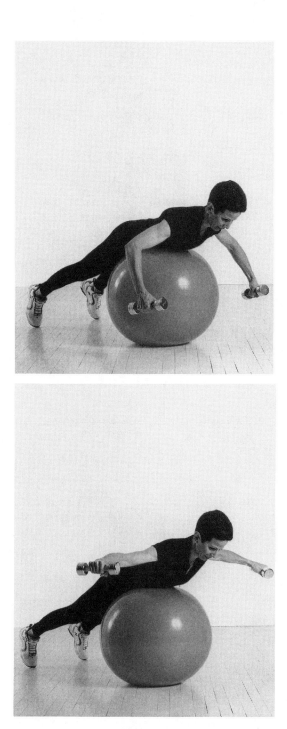

5. Rear Deltoid Fly with Ball

1. Lie on your chest on the Resist-A-Ball, your legs in a **V** position for balance with your toes on the floor.

2. Grasp one light dumbbell in each hand, with your palms facing in.

3. Start with your elbows only slightly bent, then slowly exhale as you lift your arms up and out to your sides until your palms face down.

4. Inhale as you release but don't let the dumbbells touch the floor—keep some tension.

5. Keep your toes firmly planted on the floor for balance, abdominals tucked.

6. Your head and neck maintain a neutral position while you look down.

Training tip:

If this exercise is too difficult, then position your feet against a wall for added support.

6. Dead Lift

1. Stand with your feet shoulder-width apart, toes forward, with soft knees.

2. Grasp a dumbbell in each hand, with your palms facing your thighs.

3. Pull your shoulders back and down and maintain this straight back throughout the movement. Abdominals tucked.

4. Slowly bend from the hips, not your lower back, until you feel a full stretch in your hamstrings (the back of your thighs).

5. Inhale on the way down; exhale on the way up.

6. Keep your head and chin in alignment at all times; your weight always stays on your heels.

7. Make sure that the dumbbells track straight down your legs.

8. Stop if you feel any pain in your lower back.

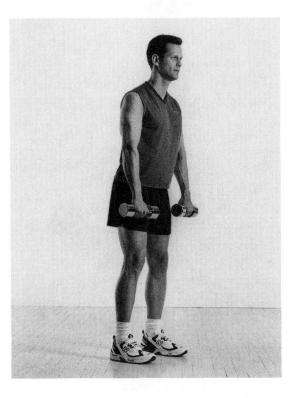

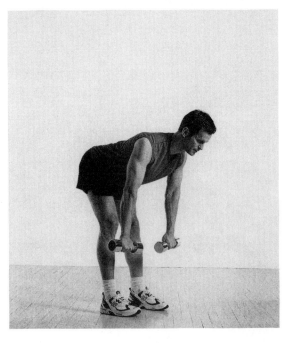

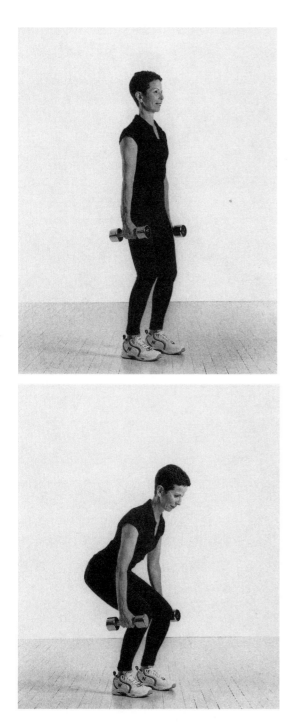

7. Squat

1. Stand with your feet shoulder-width apart, toes forward, with soft knees.

2. Grasp a dumbbell in each hand, with your palms facing your hips.

3. Pull your shoulders back and down and maintain this straight back throughout the movement. Abdominals tucked.

4. Slowly sit back into your heels and slightly bend forward to balance your body.

5. Make sure that your knees never extend over your toes.

6. Ideally, the end of the movement occurs when your hamstrings are almost parallel to the floor.

7. Inhale on the way down; exhale on the way up.

8. On the way up, really concentrate on your glutes and squeeze as you lift.

8. Stationary Lunge

1. Stand with your right foot forward, left foot back, approximately three feet apart.

2. Both toes face forward; your back heel is up at all times. Abdominals tucked.

3. Grasp a dumbbell in each hand at your sides, with your palms facing your hips. (Note: beginners may elect to start without the dumbbells.)

4. Slowly inhale as you lower your body and bend both knees.

5. Exhale as you lift and squeeze the left glute on the way up.

6. Make sure your forward right knee never passes your right toes.

7. The back knee should end approximately three inches off of the floor.

8. Repeat with left foot forward.

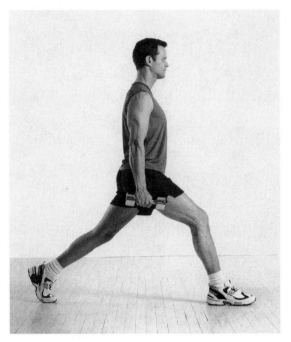

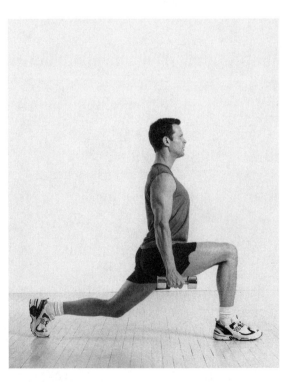

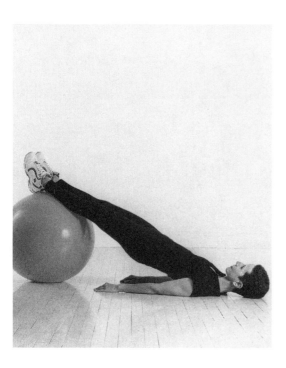

9. Hamstring Curl with Ball

1. Lie on the floor with your hands down at your sides, palms down.

2. Place your feet on the Resist-A-Ball with your toes pointed up. Keep your abdominals tucked.

3. First, lift your lower back off of the floor as you inhale, then exhale as you bend your knees, dig in your heels, and bring the ball closer to you.

4. Hold when you have curled as far as you can go, then inhale as you release.

5. Make sure to keep your back and glutes off the floor once you begin the first repetition until you complete the set.

6. Concentrate on your hamstrings as you curl in.

7. As pictured, your toes will end pointing at a more forward angle.

Training tip:

As you become more adept at performing this exercise, you may try crossing your arms over your chest to make the movement more difficult.

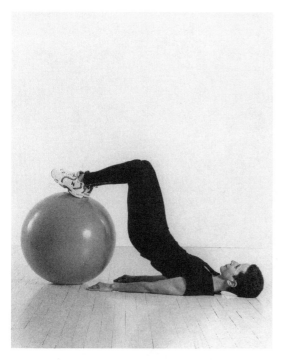

10. Abs with Ball

1. Sit on the Resist-A-Ball with your feet shoulder-width apart, toes forward. Keep your abdominals tucked.

2. Once you are balanced, cross your hands over your chest. (Note: If you are a beginner, then you may want to keep your hands on the side of the ball for balance.)

3. Slowly inhale as you lean back with a straight back.

4. In the beginning, only lean back a few inches; you will increase your range of motion as you get stronger.

5. Visualize your abdominals as a fist: As you lean back, open the fist, then clench the fist and squeeze your abdominals in as you return to starting position.

Training tip:

Beginners may want to place their toes against a wall for additional support.

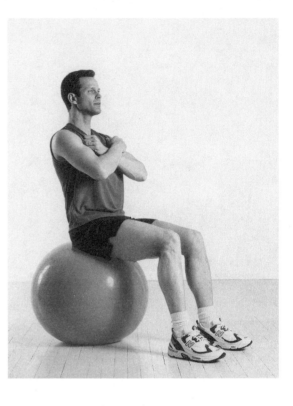

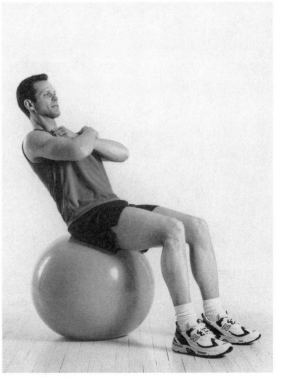

TEN EXERCISES WITH MACHINES

Perform 8 to 10 repetitions of each exercise.

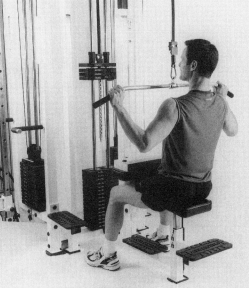

1. Lat Pulldown

1. Sit down in the lat pulldown seat and adjust the top pad so that it just comfortably touches the top of your thighs.

2. Place the weight pin at a light weight, such as 15 to 20 pounds, to start.

3. Grasp the bar with a wide overhand grip, ideally on the rubber pads as shown.

4. Start by adjusting your shoulders down and back, inhale, then exhale as you slowly pull the bar down to just below your chin.

5. As you pull down, squeeze your back muscles.

6. Slowly inhale as you release the bar to starting position, but keep your shoulders down and back and your elbows slightly bent.

7. Make sure to keep your chin and head in alignment at all times.

"I HATE TO EXERCISE"

211

2. Back Row

1. Sit on the pad and place your feet on the footrest with your toes forward.

2. Place the weight pin at a light weight, such as 10 to 15 pounds, to start.

3. Bend your knees even more as you reach for the handles of the rowing attachment. (Note: You may have to change this attachment. It's easy to do.) Be very careful not to hurt your back.

4. Make sure to tuck your abdominals as you return to starting position.

5. Set your shoulders down and back, inhale, then slowly exhale as you pull the handle back.

6. Hold when the bar is as far back as you can pull it, then inhale as you slowly release, but don't release your back muscles—keep your shoulders back.

7. Don't lean back at any time. Always finish the movement with your back perfectly straight.

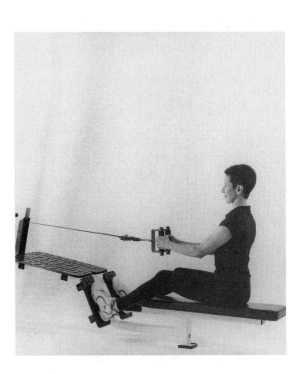

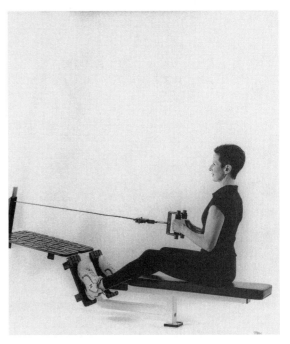

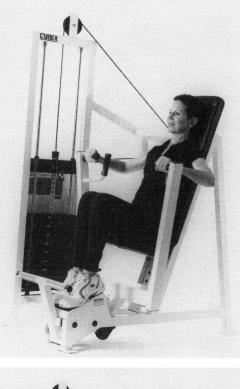

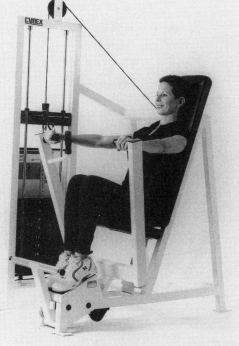

3. Chest Press

1. Sit down on the seat pad, take all the weight off, and place your hands at your sides. Keep your abdominals tucked.

2. Push the bar out with your feet, then place your hands on the pressing bars.

3. Your arms should be at shoulder height. If they are not, then adjust the seat up or down.

4. Place the weight pin at a light weight, such as 10 to 15 pounds, to start.

5. First inhale, then slowly exhale as you press the bar out.

6. Don't lock your elbows at the end; always keep them slightly bent.

7. Inhale as you release the arms back to starting position.

8. Make sure to concentrate on your chest and squeeze your pecs (chest muscles) as you push the bar out.

4. Bicep Curl

1. Find an easy curl bar in your gym. Place a light plate, such as a 2.5-pound plate, and a safety collar on each side.

2. Position yourself so that your back is straight and your upper arms comfortably rest on the pad.

3. Keep your abdominals tucked at all times.

4. Grasp the bar with your hands shoulder-width apart, right where the bar curls in, palms facing up.

5. First inhale, then exhale as you squeeze and lift up.

6. Stop when your elbows want to leave the pad; inhale on the way down.

7. Don't fully extend your arms at the beginning of the movement; maintain a slight bend.

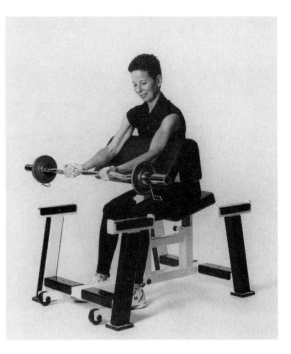

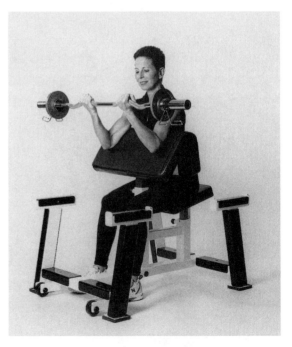

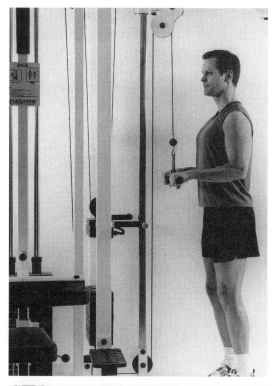

5. Tricep Pushdown

1. Place a short or long bar on a high pulley.

2. Place the weight pin at a low weight, such as 10 pounds, to start.

3. Stand in front of the bar with your feet shoulder-width apart, toes forward, and abdominals tucked.

4. Place your hands shoulder-width apart with an overhand grip, your forearms parallel to the floor.

5. First inhale, then slowly exhale as you press your arms down and squeeze your triceps in the back of each arm.

6. Inhale as you release back to starting position—forearms parallel to the floor.

7. Make sure to relax your shoulders and neck at all times; if you are lifting them up, you are using too much weight.

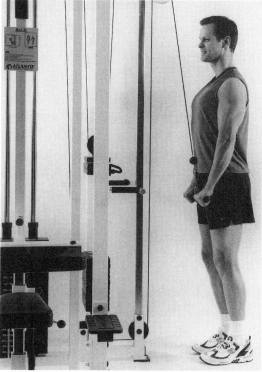

6. Leg Press

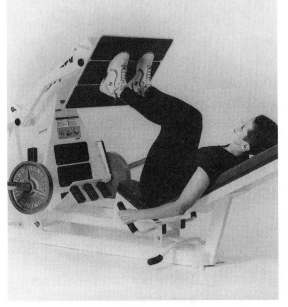

1. Place a light weight, such as a 10-pound plate, to start on each side.

2. Place your feet shoulder-width apart, toes forward.

3. Slowly exhale as you press the weight out until your legs are almost totally extended; inhale as you return.

4. Release the safety guards by pressing the side arms out. This will allow you to work a full range of motion.

5. You should lower the weight until your legs are at a 90-degree angle.

6. Make sure to keep your head on the pad at all times and relax your neck. Keep your abdominals tucked.

7. As you press up, concentrate on pushing through your heels and squeezing your glutes.

Training tip:
If you feel pressure in your neck, you might want to roll a small towel under your neck for support.

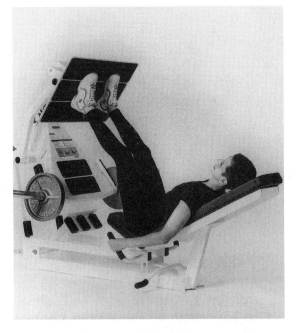

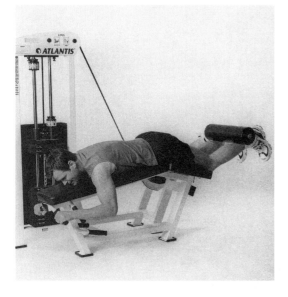

7. Hamstring Curl

1. Place the weight pin at a light weight, such as 10 pounds, to start.

2. Lie down on the hamstring curl machine with your feet underneath the roller.

3. First inhale, then slowly exhale as you curl the roller up; concentrate on your hamstrings.

4. Keep your abdominals tucked at all times to support your lower back.

5. Don't arch your back as you curl up; stay flat on the pad.

6. As you release, make sure to maintain a slight bend in the knees as pictured.

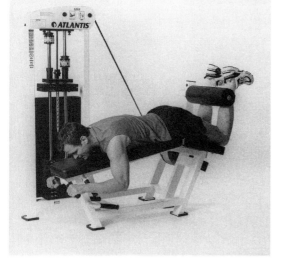

8. Hip Extension

1. Pull the weight pin out and start with the lightest weight.

2. Place the ankle cuff on your left leg—it is easy to adjust the size with the Velcro strap. Face the machine.

3. Shift your body weight onto your right leg; slightly bend both legs.

4. Hold on to the machine's handles for balance.

5. Keep your abdominals tucked and your shoulders down and back at all times.

6. Slowly press your left leg back; flex your toes up.

7. Concentrate on your left glute as you press back, though you will feel it in both glutes.

8. Repeat on the right leg.

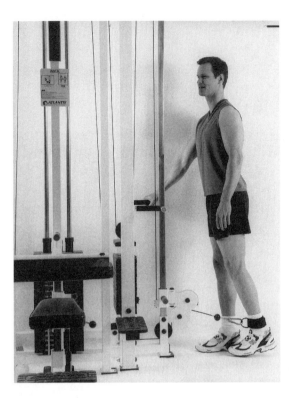

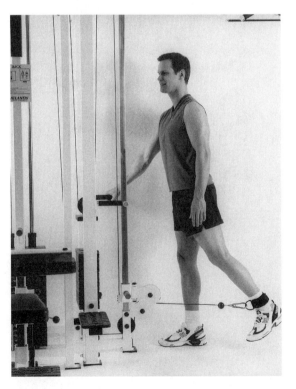

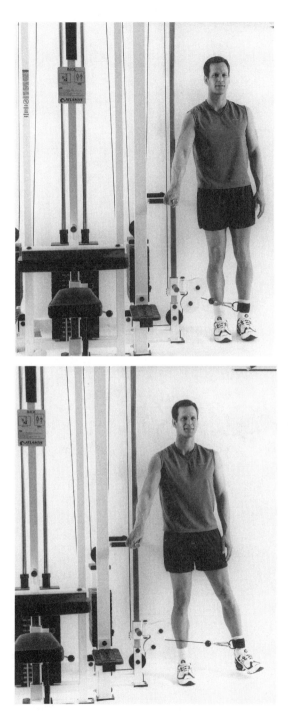

9. Hip Adduction

1. Pull the weight pin out and start with the lightest weight.

2. Place the ankle cuff on your left leg—it is easy to adjust the size with the Velcro strap. Face at a 90-degree angle from the machine.

3. Shift your body weight onto your right leg; slightly bend both legs.

4. Hold on to the machine's handles for balance.

5. Keep your abdominals tucked and your shoulders down and back at all times.

6. Slowly press your left leg out to the side; flex your toes up.

7. Concentrate on your left hip and glute as you press out, though you will feel it in both hips and glutes.

8. Repeat on the right leg.

10. The Plank

1. Begin by lying flat on the floor on your stomach.

2. First, prop your upper body up on your elbows with your head and neck in alignment.

3. Next, come up onto your knees with your toes on the floor.

4. Finally, lift up onto your toes with your abdominals tucked to support your lower back.

5. Hold for as long as you can, pause for ten seconds, then repeat two additional times for a total of three holds.

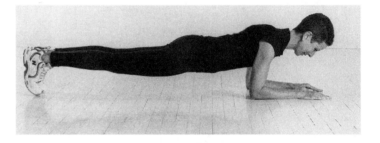

These exercises were selected and designed to provide you with a balanced, highly effective strength and resistance exercise program. Each program is equally effective in building lean muscle tissue, burning body fat, improving body composition, and, most important, boosting metabolism to lose weight.

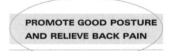

BRING THIS BOOK
TO THE GYM

Think "Back"

All three exercise programs place emphasis on the muscles in the back of the body. I do this because these muscles are generally an individual's weakest; consequently they require more attention. Consider for a moment the amount of time you spend driving, or at your desk or computer, or carrying children, grocery bags, purses, briefcases, or luggage. All of these movements and many more train your shoulders to roll forward and your back to round. This promotes poor posture and back pain. To counter these everyday activities and body patterns, I recommend that you work the large muscles of the back and the rear part of the shoulder. The same is true of the legs. We use the front of the legs, the quadriceps, every time we walk, climb a stair, or get up from a chair. When do we use the back of the legs, the hamstrings? Rarely. Therefore, more emphasis is placed on the back of the leg.

Go "Back" to the Mirror

I urge you to once again take a look at your body in a mirror. Many people, especially women, tell me, "The front of my leg is bowed out and overdeveloped, while the back is flat. My legs don't appear to be symmetrical." That is absolutely correct. Cardiovascular exercise only makes this situation worse. Walking, running, stair climbing, spinning (a killer for the front of the leg), and cycling all work the front of the leg far more than the back. In the future, cut back on the cardio and reverse this muscular imbalance by following one of my strength and resistance exercise programs.

PROMOTE GOOD POSTURE
AND RELIEVE BACK PAIN

Progression

The key to the overall effectiveness of the three *Flip the Switch* exercise programs is what is termed *progression.* Progression is an often-misunderstood concept in strength and resistance exercise programs. The following analogy will help you to better understand the concept of progression. Those of you who have studied a foreign language know that you begin with the basics. I studied French for many years (though you'd never know it by my accent—it's frightening). My first French language textbook began with the following drill:

Hello = *Bon jour*

Good-bye = *Au revoir*

My name is Jim = *Je m'appelle Jacques*

Had I continued to study that book for years and years, the only words I would have been able to speak in French would be *hello, good-bye,* and *my name is Jim.* Do you see where we are going here? To become more proficient, I had to move (or progress) on to Lesson Book Two and start to increase my vocabulary—learn more words: nouns, verbs, adjectives, and adverbs. I had to progress. Apart from actually living in the country where the language is spoken, that is the only way anyone seeking to learn a foreign language can become fluent.

You Did It Once, You Can Do It Again

Look at babies. They go through progression as they learn language. Evan, my little guy, is just eighteen months old as I write this book. In addition to loud shrieks and unintelligible words, he is just starting to clearly say "Mama," "Dada," "Oh nooooooo," "Oh baby!" "Elmo," "papo" (for popcorn), and, I will confess, "poo-poo." My wife and I certainly hope that his vocabulary will increase. How will it grow? Progression. He'll hear more words; he'll learn; he'll progress.

You Succeed When You Fail

Remember my discussion of what occurs when you fatigue a muscle and it ultimately fails? That "failure" then stimulates the muscle to grow so that it can perform the exercise with greater ability. With strength and resistance exercise, you basically succeed when you fail. What happens when you stop challenging the muscle? The muscle will *not* be prompted to grow, change, and burn more calories. At best you would maintain your existing lean muscle, and don't forget that with age muscle begins to atrophy; properly employed strength and resistance exercise will reverse this process. You need to constantly keep progressing by applying one or a combination of the following techniques to your strength and resistance exercise program.

Progression Technique 1: Increase the Weight or Tension

The simplest way to apply progression is to increase the resistance involved in the exercise. This is accomplished by:

- *For exercise program 1,* the SPRI Xertube, Xering, and Resist-A-Ball workout, you have two options. First, you can move farther away from the tube attachment point. An example would be to place the ball farther away from the door for the back row and the rear deltoid fly. By doing this, you will increase the resistance of the exercise. Second, you can go up in tension. From easiest to hardest, the Xertubes and Xerings progress in the following order: yellow, green, red, blue, and purple.

- *For exercise program 2,* the free weight and Resist-A-Ball workout, moving to a heavier weight constitutes progression. If you begin with five-pound dumbbells, move up to eight pounds. From eight pounds, which is the intermediate level, advance to ten. I recommend that inexperienced exercisers start with three to five pounds of weight. If you're experienced but "rusty," go for five pounds. Just don't be afraid to ultimately increase to the twelve-, fifteen-, and twenty-pound dumbbells (or more) for certain exercises.

- *For exercise program 3,* the machine workout, increasing the weight pin by the smallest increment constitutes progression. Most newer machines allow you to increase the weight by as little as 2.5 pounds or they come with a small 2.5-pound plate that you can place on top of the weight stack.

The key to successful progression of all three programs is to increase the weight or tension by the smallest increment available.

You may notice that performing all the repetitions with the new weight or tension may be too difficult. In that instance, do as many repetitions as you can with the higher weight or tension, then drop down to the former weight or tension to finish your set.

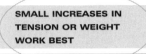

SMALL INCREASES IN TENSION OR WEIGHT WORK BEST

Never try to jump up in tube tension or weight too quickly. Doing so can lead to an injury. I want you to believe in yourself and gain confidence, but don't be unrealistic. Always use the smallest increment for safe and effective progression.

Progression Technique 2: Increase the Repetitions

This option is quite easy to apply. Simply increase the number of repetitions. Do note that the maximum benefits of your strength and resistance program are derived by performing no more than twelve repetitions of any one exercise. Very recent research indicates that the optimal building of lean muscle tissue occurs in a set of eight to ten repetitions. I want you to derive the most out of the time you've allotted to exercise. Therefore, I want you to keep the reps on the low side. Remember what I wrote earlier: It is not the amount of time you devote to exercise that makes the difference, it is the way you exercise. Keep the reps low and the weight or tension resistance up. That's what gets the job done.

High Reps, Low Weight versus Low Reps, High Weight

This is a subject that I know confuses many people. For years, the fitness industry led the consumer to believe that low reps, high weight was best for building muscle, and high reps, low weight was best for "toning." We know from my discussion on page 173 that there really is no such thing as "toning." That so-called toned look occurs when lean muscle tissue is increased and fat is burned. That goal, building muscle and burning fat, optimally occurs with a low repetition, high weight protocol.

PERFORM NO MORE THAN 12 REPETITIONS OF EACH EXERCISE

Progression Technique 3: Increase the Sets

Each of my three illustrated exercise programs recommends that you begin with one set of each exercise, each set consisting of no more than twelve repetitions, optimally only eight to ten reps. Most research indicates that 85 to 90 percent of the benefits of strength and resistance training occurs in the first set when performed to failure. So, if you work until failure, one set is all that you need. However, those of you who wish to do more than one set of each exercise should go ahead, if you have the time, discipline, and are willing to push yourself. And those of you who adopt the one-set protocol should not be concerned. Doing additional sets at this point in your program is by no means necessary. I included this option because it is one of the elements of exercise progression.

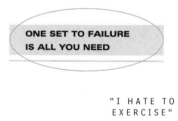

ONE SET TO FAILURE
IS ALL YOU NEED

Progression Technique 4: Slow Down

Slowing the speed of the exercise is one of my favorite progression methods that I use with clients. On page 183, I urged you to use a three count on the exertion, or the contraction of the muscle, a one-count hold, and a three count on the release. For many of you, this will be challenging in the beginning. But after you can perform twelve repetitions with ease, you may decide to simply increase the time that it takes to perform each repetition. You can go from a three count to a four count, a four count to a five count, and so on up to ten.

Now You Tell Me

You are probably asking yourself, "Why didn't you tell me to go this slowly in the first place?" My answer to that question is, "Learning strength and resistance exercise is not easy." As I said earlier, it

GO SLOW FOR FASTER RESULTS

Research conducted by Wayne Westcott in 1993 and again in 1999 separated individuals who previously were not performing strength and resistance exercise into two groups. The first group performed ten repetitions of each exercise, spending several seconds on each repetition, and the other group performed five repetitions, but spent a total of fourteen seconds on each repetition. The slow lifters were moving at half the speed of the other group. Over a period of eight to ten weeks, the slow lifters gained 50 percent more strength than the control group. What this clearly indicates is that slow is the way to go when performing strength and resistance exercises.

requires you to concentrate and use your body in an unfamiliar manner. The key to this program is adherence and consistency. At the start of the physical-exercise component of flipping, I didn't want to use a technique so difficult that you would become discouraged. I want you to feel that you can do the exercise program, master the technique, then apply the necessary progression for even greater results. Trust me, you will be progressing in no time and when you do, you will clearly see the results of your hard work. Don't forget, you have already visualized those results in your mind. Now you will actually start to see them on your body, and that will motivate you more than you can imagine.

Progression Technique 5: Add Instability

Adding instability is somewhat more difficult than the first four progression techniques. When I say "add instability," I mean that you should use a Resist-A-Ball from SPRI Products rather than a weight bench, or go from standing on both legs to standing on one leg when performing an exercise.

First, let's look at the Resist-A-Ball. I included the ball in exercise programs 1 and 2 because it is a highly versatile and comfortable piece of equipment. It naturally incorporates the technique of progression. There is a considerable difference between sitting on a bench or a chair and sitting on the ball when performing an exercise. The bench and chair are stable; they don't move. Balance is not a problem. The ball, on the other hand, moves. It is an unstable surface. If you shift your weight, you have to compensate for this shift by using other muscles to keep your balance on the ball. If you don't, you can easily fall.

Therefore, when you perform exercises on the ball, you are challenging your body much more than would be the case if the exercise were performed on a stable surface like an exercise bench or a chair.

So, to add significant progression to your exercise program, sit on the ball when possible. You will also be working more of your "core" (abdominals and lower back), which I touched upon earlier. You get the benefits of strengthening both the muscle you are isolating and your core as well—two benefits for the energy output of one exercise.

You can also bring progression to your exercise program by standing on one leg instead of two. For example, a simple bicep curl (see page 194) is dramatically changed when you stand on only one leg. Your entire center of gravity is altered. The leg you are standing on now requires more energy to support the weight of your entire body. Your abdominals and lower back—your core—have to jump in to assist the body to stay in alignment. You are further challenging your body, which is the whole idea behind progression, resulting in increased muscular strength and size.

You can even take this one step further and exercise with a SPRI Xerdisc, which you can see at my website, www.jimkaras.com. This is a small inflatable disc that looks like a flying saucer. By using the disc, which costs about $30, you bring instability into the exercise. Here is how it can be used:

How to Use the SPRI Xerdisc

- Stand on one leg on the Xerdisc. Just stand on the disc and apply progression to your exercise routine. Try it while watching television, even for a minute or two on each leg. I promise you will feel it.

- Stand on the Xerdisc. You can use it under your front foot when performing lunges or under one foot when performing squats. Try it. You will really feel the difference.

- When performing push-ups, place one hand on the Xerdisc and the other hand on the floor. Perform five or six repetitions with it under the right hand, then switch to the left. You will dramatically feel the difference in your chest.

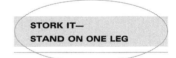
GET ON THE BALL TO NATURALLY INCORPORATE PROGRESSION

STORK IT— STAND ON ONE LEG

THE PUSH-UP

While I have not included a photograph of a push-up in any of my three exercise programs, performing push-ups can be an effective way to challenge and work the upper body, particularly the chest, shoulders, and arms. To do a push-up:

1. Place your hands shoulder-width apart, fingers spread.

2. If you are a beginner, balance on your knees. If you feel stronger, lift up on your toes.

3. Keep your abdominals tucked at all times to support your lower back.

4. Slowly inhale as you lower down to two inches above the floor; exhale as you press back up.

5. Make sure your chin goes just over your fingertips.

6. Concentrate on your chest at all times, especially as you press up.

7. If you fatigue early on your toes, then drop down to your knees to complete the set of eight to ten repetitions.

• When performing classic abdominal crunches place the Xerdisc in the small of your back to add stability and really challenge your abs.

Let's Fail

I already raised the issue of "failure" while exercising, and I would like to clarify that point a bit further. Your body passes through three stages as you perform a set of strength and resistance repetitions.

The Three Stages of Strength and Resistance Exercise

Stage 1: Working Repetitions

When you first begin a strength and resistance exercise set, the weight you train with should be challenging, but not so challenging that it is impossible for you to perform the exercise. You are performing what I refer to as the "working repetitions." Working repetitions should be performed with terrific form, relaxed breathing, and good posture. They should consist of five to six repetitions.

Stage 2: Fatigue

As you perform your working repetitions, the exercise becomes more difficult with each repetition. You will feel a slight "burn" in the muscle and experience some difficulty maintaining correct form. What's happening is that the muscle you are using is "fatiguing" and is beginning to experience difficulty performing additional repetitions. Stage 2, fatigue, will last for two to three repetitions.

YOU SUCCEED WHEN YOU FAIL

Stage 3: Failure

As you are in the last repetitions of fatigue, you find that you are no longer able to move the band, weight, or machine: Your muscles are in failure. Congratulations! Congratulations on failing? That's right, failure is the goal. This is one of the few activities in life where you succeed when you fail.

The Catalyst to Growth

The fatigue and the resulting failure are the catalysts for muscle growth. This is the process that builds lean muscle tissue and leads to improved muscularity, reduced body fat, and the increase in your metabolism. To repeat: If you don't hit *failure,* then you are *not* getting the job done and building the lean muscle tissue that you need to succeed at weight loss.

Feeling Plateaued Out?

Over the years, many people have told me that their body hit a "plateau." This is not the case. Their body hasn't hit a plateau, their exercise program has. Unfortunately, most individuals perform the same exercise routine for weeks, months, or even years without ever applying progression. Progression is essential to your continued success at weight loss. Progression is the key to your staying flipped.

Mix It Up

Now, as you are determining which exercise program to follow, you may be wondering, "Can I mix and match the three exercise programs? Can I do part with the tubing, part with free weights, and when I have the time, go to a club to do the machines?" Absolutely. I designed these three programs for you to introduce you to strength and resistance exercise, or to fine-tune your program if you are already doing this style of exercise. You may ultimately mix and match these programs any way you wish: part gym, part home, part office. You may find yourself doing one of the two home exercise programs on some weekdays and the machine workout at a club on the weekends. The choice is yours. This is possible because of our next essential component to your exercise plan—documentation.

Documentation: Record Your Progression

I recommend that you keep a detailed training log for your exercise plan. (For each of my three exercise programs, you'll find a blank form you can photocopy in the back of this book.) Here are suggested headings that you should complete:

EXERCISE	BAND/WEIGHT	REPETITIONS	DATE

For the lat pulldown exercise in Program A, you would record:

EXERCISE	BAND/WEIGHT	REPETITIONS	DATE
Lat Pulldown w/ball	Red	12	1/04

The log provides you with the documentation you need for progression: a record of what you've done and what you need to do. Once you have completed a log you may choose to file it away for future reference. Then you can look back and see how much you have accomplished with this plan.

The training log, similar to the time-log journal, the budget, and the food diary, forces you to look at what you are or are not doing in black and white. If you find that you are not seeing all the positive results associated with flipping, you may realize that you are not progressing with your exercise plan.

All of my staff, including myself, maintain training logs for our clients. If you have ever worked with or are presently working with a personal fitness trainer who does not maintain a training log, then you should explore hiring another trainer who keeps records of your work. The training log may be the single most essential motivational/instructional tool when it comes to effective strength and resistance exercise.

PUTTING IT ALL TOGETHER TO FLIP

- Classic dieting alone will not take the weight off or keep it off.

- Strength and resistance exercise overrides the body's resistance to classic dieting.

- Strength and resistance boosts the body's metabolism twenty-four hours a day, seven days a week, 365 days a year.

- Strength and resistance exercise preserves and creates lean muscle tissue, which burns more calories on a daily basis to maintain itself than fat tissue.

- Strength and resistance exercise effectively manipulates the Balance of Energy Equation to permanently achieve weight loss.

- Cardiovascular exercise alone cannot achieve permanent weight-loss results.

- Allocate 25 percent of your exercise time to cardiovascular exercise and 75 percent of your time to strength and resistance exercise.

- Don't be intimidated by strength and resistance exercise no matter what your age, weight, or gender.

- Everyone was a beginner at one time. Just keep saying, "If they can do it, so can I. If they can do it, so can I."

9 "I'm a Woman"

Sitting in front of me is a female client who has achieved success in almost every area of her life. She may be an attorney, a corporate executive, a homemaker, or a charity fund-raiser. It doesn't matter. What matters to her is that at this point in her life she feels she is not complete. She feels she is failing. Why would someone who is so outwardly successful possess such feelings? Well, for starters, with each succeeding year she has experienced a degree of weight gain. Each year a little more weight accumulates and the closer she is to approaching fifty, the faster that weight gain increases. As she speaks, I see the emotion. I see the despair and I note phrases such as: "Why is this happening to me? My old dieting tricks don't work anymore. I feel like I am losing control of myself with every pound I gain. I am looking older. My husband has gained a little bit of weight, but not nearly as much as I have. It's just not fair being a woman." My response is always the following: "This doesn't have to happen. Yes, it gets harder as you age; yes, weight loss is harder for women than for men; but, yes, you can lose the weight and regain control of your body. I will help you help yourself. Believe me. Now let's get to work."

"REMEMBER,
GINGER ROGERS
DID EVERYTHING
FRED ASTAIRE
DID, BUT SHE DID
IT BACKWARDS
AND IN HIGH
HEELS."
—FAITH WHITTLESEY

Yes, weight loss is harder for women than it is for men. However, this does not mean that weight loss is impossible for women. Through my books, lectures, workshops, and articles, I have helped hundreds, if not thousands, of women lose weight.

To properly examine the excuse "I'm a woman," it is necessary to first look at the physiological barriers to flipping the switch and then explore the difficult psychological issues. I want you to understand how your body and mind differ from those of a man (given, of course, the obvious) and how these differences relate to weight loss. Yes, you will get your body back, and if you never liked that body in the first place, you will now. Once again, I have done it for others—I will do the same for you.

The Physiological Barriers to Flipping the Switch

To begin the physiological analysis, we need to revisit the Balance of Energy Equation and apply it this time solely to women:

BALANCE OF ENERGY EQUATION

| ENERGY IN | (CALORIES) − | ENERGY OUT | (METABOLISM AND ACTIVITY) = | BODY WEIGHT |

Yes, we've seen how this equation applies to both men and women. However, six physiological factors that relate specifically to women strongly influence the outcome of the equation:

Physiological Factor 1

Women must monitor their *calories in* much more than men because they do not expend as many *calories out* through metabolism and activity. Why? Because most women are smaller. This may also help you to understand why some of your taller friends do not struggle with weight loss as much as your shorter friends. In general, the larger the individual:

- The more calories his or her body burns at rest. The larger the body mass, the more that body's internal organs have to work to properly function and service that larger mass. These metabolic functions require more calories.

MOST WOMEN ARE SMALLER THAN MEN, SO THEY BURN FEWER CALORIES

- The more calories his or her body burns during activity and exercise, because it's moving a greater mass through space.

Physiological Factor 2

Women possess more body fat and less lean muscle tissue than men. Why?

- First, female reproductive organs and breasts increase the percentage of a woman's essential body fat ("essential" meaning the minimum amount required to function properly). Women require 12 percent essential body fat; men require only 3 percent.

- Second, both men and women produce the male hormone testosterone, but men produce more of this hormone than women. Testosterone enhances muscle building. As I stated in the previous chapter, men have twenty to thirty times the muscle-building potential of women. Maintaining and possessing a greater ability to build muscle enables men to burn more calories through their metabolism than women. Keep in mind that I stress throughout this book that muscle is the body's most metabolically active tissue. It burns between thirty-five and fifty calories per pound per day. Fat only burns 2 calories each day.

Even if a man and a woman are the same age, height, and weight, the man almost *always* possesses a higher metabolism and burns more calories than the woman because of this difference in body composition.

All of the women who are concerned that they will get big and bulky as a result of strength and resistance training should realize that in my fifteen years of experience, I have *never* seen a woman who followed my plan "bulk up." Remember, bulkiness you may have observed in fitness magazines or at your local health club or gym is likely the result of an excessive exercise regime or the use of dangerous steroids and supplements. It's actually quite difficult even for men to bulk up without the use of these products. You won't get bulky with strength and resistance exercise. On the contrary, you will become lean and thin.

Physiological Factor 3

Women have menstrual cycles. A woman's menstrual cycle produces a myriad of physical and mental factors that occur throughout each and every month. They include:

- *Physical bloating.* During menstruation, and for some during ovulation, hormone changes may cause a woman's water balance to shift. This shift can cause a woman to experience water retention that is both noticeable visually and physically uncomfortable.

YOU'LL LOOK LONG AND LEAN—NOT BULKY— WITH STRENGTH AND RESISTANCE EXERCISE

- *Food cravings.* As hormonal changes occur throughout the month, many women feel cravings for certain foods, many of which include salt, fat, or sugar.

- *Emotional highs and lows.* Many women feel that their emotions are heightened during menstruation and/or ovulation. This can lead them to overeat as they react to these mood swings.

- *Lack of energy.* A sizable percentage of women experience a noticeable lack of energy at certain times of the month, and their desire to exercise diminishes. Ironically, the overwhelming emotional and physical benefits derived from exercise would make most women feel better at this time.

Don't forget, women experience this on a monthly basis, some in a more severe form than others. This response can also change throughout life, and frequently childbirth will alter a woman's cycle and its symptoms. I have had women in their forties say to me, "I never used to experience the emotional highs and lows and the food cravings my friends talk about. Now I see what they mean. I feel as if I am doing battle every month with my body. Just thinking about my period makes me want to cry. What can I do?" In order to gain a clearer understanding of your feelings, please complete the following two sentences in the spaces provided at right. I usually provide you with my response to these emotional exercises, but I've elected to pass—for obvious reasons.

The Defensive Strategy

The more aware you are of the physical and emotional changes that occur during certain times of the month, the better you can deal with the consequences. And,

"I'M A WOMAN"—

When I have my period and/or during ovulation, I physically feel . . .

_____

_____

_____

_____

_____

When I have my period and/or during ovulation, I emotionally feel . . .

_____

_____

_____

_____

_____

_____

if you have a good idea when these shifts will occur, you can plan a defensive strategy to minimize your reactions. That strategy can include setting a date with a good friend to exercise and have dinner the day before your period is due to begin. For a great many women, the day before their period arrives is generally the "worst" day of the month. Another strategy might be to plan a day out of the house, working, shopping, or running errands when you know that sticking around the house may lead you to overeat (I know it does for me and I don't have menstrual cycles). You might plan to get your hair cut, or have a manicure or massage, something that makes you feel good about you and lifts your spirits. Blasting music in my car when I am feeling low and alone (I get so tired of listening to *Elmo, Beauty and the Beast,* and *Madeline*) makes me feel better. These tips may sound mundane, but they can help. You're thinking in advance. You might not have a "perfect" eating and exercise day, but you could minimize if not eliminate the damage to your flip.

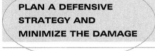

PLAN A DEFENSIVE
STRATEGY AND
MINIMIZE THE DAMAGE

Physiological Factor 4

Women bear children. Many women who go through childbirth experience the following:

- *Weight gain issues.* Naturally, it is essential that a woman gain weight to carry a healthy child. After delivery and the subsequent loss of weight that results from the birth, most women still require a weight loss of anywhere between ten and fifty pounds. For some women, this may be the first time they have had to address weight loss. For others, it may be the beginning of the Slow-Gainer pattern of weight gain.

- *Difficult delivery.* The act of childbirth can be traumatic for the mother both emotionally and physically. In addition, according to Frederic D. Frigoletto Jr., M.D., chief of obstetrics at Massachusetts General Hospital in Boston, "If you're having your first baby, there's a one in four or five chance that you'll have a C-section." A cesarean section requires more time for recovery. Many women are exhausted from a long labor, which is not only physically depleting but mentally exhausting as well. It can lead to depression, which results in overeating and reduced physical activity and exercise.

- *Hormonal changes.* Almost from the moment of conception, a pregnant woman's body goes through significant hormonal changes. These changes can cause nausea; morning, afternoon, and evening sickness (many women have told me, "Whoever named this morning sickness never carried a child—I was sick around the clock"); overeating; depression; and sleep deprivation, to name but a few. Pregnancy can be an extremely difficult time for a woman, whose distress may be further exacerbated by friends and family who say that pregnancy should be the most joyous, wonderful time in a woman's life. For many women, this is anything but the case.

- *Breast-feeding issues.* Breast feeding normally is a wonderful experience for mother and child. It can lead to a deep bonding between the two. In addition, breast-feeding is known to enhance the ability of the uterus to contract back to normal size after delivery. However, breast-feeding can be a frustrating time when either the mother is not producing enough milk or the baby is having a difficult time adapting to the challenge of breast-feeding—sometimes both of these factors are present. I've heard numerous new moms say over the years that they felt they "failed" because they could not continue to breast-feed. Of course they haven't failed, but an emotional issue such as this can lead to further depression and stress.

  Breast-feeding can make weight loss even more difficult, since a woman needs additional calories (approximately 300) each day to manufacture milk. But breast-feeding itself can burn approximately 500 additional calories a day. Therefore, you could actually be creating a 200-calorie deficit each day. In seventeen and a half days you could lose a pound (17.5 days times 200 calories equals 3,500 calories, or one pound). Just be very careful to consume only an additional 300 calories a day.

- *Sleep deprivation. Parenting* magazine reports that "nearly one quarter of sleep-deprived moms scored high on depression tests." Take a moment to flip back to page 78 in Chapter 4, "'I Don't Have the Energy.'" The sleep deprivation that occurs in many new mothers can be detrimental to physical health and emotional well-being. For some, it can be the start of an ongoing struggle to get adequate sleep. Please make a note of this issue. Look back at your time-log journal from Chapter 3. Nap if necessary; try to get into bed even a few minutes earlier each night. Make sleep a priority. Being well rested, both physically and mentally, is one of the keys to successful flipping as well as successful parenting. And remember, the early months of interrupted sleep eventually do come to an end.

- *Postpartum depression.* The majority of postpartum depression cases are frequently far less severe than what we have read about or seen depicted in the media. But the reality is that many women do go through some degree of depression after giving birth. This seems to be especially true for first-time moms, though it can occur with each subsequent birth. The fantasy of family life with baby is quite different from the reality. Managing a newborn is tough. Years ago, women didn't openly discuss how difficult it was to manage a new baby. They probably didn't talk about it because nobody asked. It was a woman's job. Period. The "accepted" philosophy of the time was that all women loved having babies. Having a baby and a life as a homemaker was what young girls were told was the proper career choice. Not to aspire to such a life was considered outside "the norm."

Today, the situation is very different. For one thing, economic realities often dictate that most women will work outside the home. Many will do so because they desire a career. Regardless of the reason, a great many mothers working outside the home and considerable numbers of mothers working inside the home will experience feelings of depression and anxiety about what they are doing. Those who work outside the home may miss their children and worry that they aren't providing them with enough attention during their formative years. Those who stay at home may feel "cheated," perhaps unfulfilled. Both groups will feel societal pressure to be a "super mom," a world-class homemaker, a success in her career, and a compassionate soul mate to her spouse or partner, as well as being charming, attractive, sexy, and, yes, "slim." This is

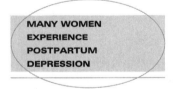

MANY WOMEN EXPERIENCE POSTPARTUM DEPRESSION

a difficult job description to fill. Add to all of this a baby who won't sleep through the night and those extra twenty pounds that just don't seem to vanish and you can quickly understand why many women experience a postpartum funk.

All this can be even worse for a single mother. The responsibility of raising a child alone plus the economic burden can be overwhelming. I applaud the single mother and realize how difficult her role is. The same sort of pressure is rarely put on a dad. His "super dad" issues tend to be more along economic lines.

- *Weight loss.* Have you ever heard a woman say that she left the hospital after delivery in the jeans she wore before she was pregnant? I have. Guess what? It's a total lie. First of all, it's impossible for a woman's uterus to contract enough for her to be able to wear tight jeans. Second, a woman's hips shift to make room for the expanding uterus and the growing fetus. It would be impossible for the hips to return to their original position in a few days. Third, unless the mother did not gain an appropriate amount of weight during pregnancy, it would be virtually impossible to lose all the excess pregnancy weight in only a few days.

The Baby versus the Behavior

Each and every new mom has to deal with weight loss. As I stated earlier in this chapter, for some women, this may be the first time they have had to address their eating and exercise programs in detail. The majority of these women now have to deal with losing the weight they gained during pregnancy in addition to the ten, twenty, thirty, or more pounds they wanted to lose *before* becoming pregnant. What prior to pregnancy seemed difficult, now appears totally impossible. Some just give up. They throw up their hands and decide to just forget weight loss and live with their present body. I have frequently heard the following remark in initial client consultations: "The baby just ruined my body—it will never be the same." This is sometimes stated years, if not decades, after the baby was born. Obviously, men do not have to deal with this difficult physical and emotional reality.

DON'T BLAME THE BABY

"I'M A WOMAN"

After I delivered my baby, I physically felt . . .

_____

_____

_____

_____

_____

_____

_____

After I delivered my baby, I emotionally felt . . .

_____

_____

_____

_____

_____

_____

_____

I want those of you who find yourself in a similar situation to complete the sentences in the spaces provided at left.

I have found from working with clients that it is so important to understand these thoughts and feelings and to put the experience of childbirth into perspective. A few years ago I saw a relative at my grandmother's funeral whom I had not seen in years. She had gained a considerable amount of weight. Before a "hello," "how are you?" or "nice to see you," or an expression of sympathy regarding my grandmother's death, she blurted out, "My kids just ruined my body." The youngest of her kids is about twenty-five years old! Obviously, my occupation makes her nervous, but her outburst indicates that she is hanging on to a decades-old pregnancy as an excuse for her present state. Once again, this is not what I want for you. Women have been giving birth since the beginning of the human race and millions and probably billions of them regained the body they desired. Trust me, this is your future as well. Read on and keep believing in your power as an agent of change.

Physiological Factor 5

Women go through menopause. As a woman enters menopause, she will begin to experience some of the following:

- _An accelerated loss of lean muscle tissue._ As previously noted, the average person, male or female, loses between one-half and seven-tenths of a pound of muscle each year. As a woman approaches menopause, she begins to lose muscle at almost twice that rate. This diminishment of muscle causes her body composition to change _and_ she experiences a significant drop in her metabolism, or daily caloric burning. This explains some

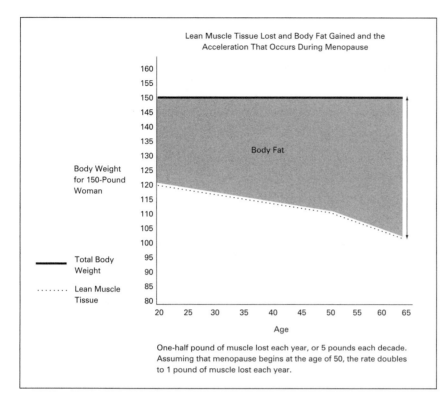

Lean Muscle Tissue Lost and Body Fat Gained and the
Acceleration That Occurs During Menopause

One-half pound of muscle lost each year, or 5 pounds each decade.
Assuming that menopause begins at the age of 50, the rate doubles
to 1 pound of muscle lost each year.

of the weight gain that many women experience at this time and thereafter. Take a look at the above graph and, assuming menopause occurs at age fifty, how the loss of muscle accelerates.

• *A thickening of the midsection of the body.* This occurs because the lipoprotein lipase begins to redirect body fat to a woman's midsection. Many women start to gain body fat in their abdominal area, contrary to their previous pattern of body fat gain, which had been primarily confined to the hips, thighs, and arms. Additionally, the female hormone estrogen diminishes with menopause, and women start to experience more of a male pattern of body fat gain. This compositional shift "around the middle" can occur even in individuals who have not gained any weight.

At this point, many women express the feeling that they have lost control of their body. Their old dieting tricks don't work, their clothes don't fit, the scale simply refuses to budge, and emotionally they begin to feel overwhelmed.

"I'M A WOMAN"

During or after menopause, I physically feel/felt . . .

_____

_____

_____

_____

_____

_____

_____

During or after menopause, I emotionally feel/felt . . .

_____

_____

_____

_____

_____

_____

_____

_____

This is not inevitable. I repeat, this is not inevitable. There is a cure for that "thickening" in the midsection, or intra-abdominal tissue. Yes, research has shown that strength and resistance exercise, not cardiovascular exercise, significantly reduces abdominal fat in the midsection in healthy older women.

If you have gone through or are presently in menopause, I want you to complete the sentences in the spaces provided at left. Of all the factors I have discussed, I have found that menopause was the principal catalyst for weight gain in many women, combined with a pronounced shift in body composition. During this period in their lives, many women have said that they physically feel a lack of energy, have trouble sleeping, which I have stressed is one of the keys to a successful flip, and sometimes lose interest in sex. It's almost as if they are doing battle with their body. Emotionally, they feel more depressed, anxious, and cheated. "Why is this happening to me?" so many lament. "Why do I feel as if my body is no longer my own?" Only you can determine how menopause has affected you and your ability to flip.

Menopause: The Perfect Time to Flip

There are positive aspects to menopause. It represents what can be a liberating passage in a woman's life. You no longer have to deal with a monthly period and its accompanying bloat, mood swings, and depression, nor with birth control and pregnancy issues. Menopause should not be looked upon as a death sentence, as some women have described it. Unfortunately, for years the media generally depicted menopause as the beginning of the "end," a time of hot flashes, emotional outbursts, and tears. Today, we know that does not have to be the case. The better you understand the physical and psychological factors associated with menopause, the better you will be able to cope with it successfully. Menopause can be the time to take control of your body—the ideal time to flip the switch.

ARE YOU DOING BATTLE WITH YOUR BODY?

Physiological Factor 6

As humans age, a loss of bone occurs. According to a new study, "roughly half of all women aged 50 or older have either low bone mass or osteoporosis *and don't know it.*" The following factors can contribute to low bone mass and osteoporosis:

- *Women start their lives with less bone mass than men.* Therefore, once bone loss occurs, women lose a greater percentage of that bone than men.

- *Excessive dieting in adolescence.* Dieting in young people can cause bones to develop improperly. Later in life, the fact that the bone was not properly formed contributes to a more rapid diminishment of bone mass.

- *Age-related loss of bone mass.* During the first five to seven years after menopause, women lose as much as 20 percent of their bone mass. This is in addition to the loss that occurred from the age of twenty until menopause if you had not been performing strength and resistance excercise.

- *Calcium deficiency.* Calcium is an essential mineral for reducing the risk of bone mass loss, osteoporosis, and fractures. From the ages of nineteen through fifty, adults need 1,000 milligrams of calcium a day, according to the National Academy of Science's Institute of Medicine. After age fifty-one, you need 1,200 milligrams. Postmenopausal women not taking estrogen need 1,500 milligrams, according to doctors at Harvard Medical School, as do all adults over age sixty-five. Pregnant or lactating women also have special needs (ranging from 1,000 to 1,300 milligrams, depending on age). Check with your doctor to get the latest calcium guidelines.

WOMEN BATTLE OSTEOPOROSIS

According to the April 2001 issue of *Medicine & Science in Sports & Exercise,* "bone mineral density is affected by genetics, exercise, hormonal status and nutrition. Although genetics appears to have the greatest impact, exercise can modify the peak bone mass a person acquires or maintains."

Bone expert C. Conrad Johnston of the Indiana University School of Medicine describes osteoporosis simply by stating that "people think bone is structurally like steel, but it's actually an active organ. Osteoclasts are cells that keep digging holes in the bone, while osteoblasts keep filling them back in." Therefore, you can control the rate at which you lose and regain bone through strength and resistance exercise and proper nutrition.

Numerous variables can halt or slow the loss of bone and perform the function of the osteoblasts. One of these is consuming the following foods:

Foods That Slow Bone Loss

NUTRIENT	MILLIGRAMS	FOODS
Calcium	1,000–1,200	Dark green leafy vegetables, broccoli, canned salmon and sardines, yogurt and cottage cheese
Vitamin C	200	Citrus fruits, strawberries, kiwi, papaya, mango, broccoli, tomatoes, potatoes, cantaloupe
Vitamin D	700–1,000	Vitamin D–fortified milk
Vitamin K	90–120	Brussels sprouts, broccoli, dark green leafy vegetables

Yes, women can win what I call "the battle of the bone." All that's required is knowledge and attention.

The Psychological Barriers to Flipping the Switch

This section discusses some of the psychological barriers women voice in an attempt to explain why they have had to struggle to successfully flip the switch.

Mothers and Daughters

During the past fifteen years in the weight-loss profession, I have listened to many poignant accounts of the relationship between mothers and daughters. Body image, whether of the mother, the daughter, or both, is frequently the most emotional of all mother-daughter issues. In writing this book, I interviewed dozens of women who represented a cross section of American women and asked them what influence their mothers had on their body image and weight issues in general. It surprised me how common the themes were. Here is what I found.

Are You Sure You Want to Eat "That"?

A large group of mothers made their daughters' body weight an issue very early in their children's lives. Some of these mothers were insecure about their own body image and simply projected that image onto their daughters. Some believed that their daughters would be happier and more successful if they lived "leaner." Others were perhaps living vicariously through their daughters. These daughters, possibly you among them, became a product of that programming.

Thelma and Marie

Marie Brenner is a wonderful friend, a client, and the author of numerous bestselling books, including *Great Dames*. Marie is a contributing writer-at-large for *Vanity Fair*. She wrote the feature piece that was ultimately made into the movie *The Insider*, starring Russell Crowe. You've probably read or seen some of her work. Marie is a great personal and professional success, with one exception that she is willing to share. She has agreed to "go public" with her relationship to food, her body image, and her early programming from her mother. Her story and insights are fascinating. What struck me most was when she said to me, "My mother is my metabolism." I asked what exactly she meant by this comment. She said, "How I feel about my body, my body weight, and my issues with food is controlled by my mother. She is my metabolism." (For the record, Marie's mom, Thelma, passed away years ago.)

SOMETIMES MOTHER DOESN'T KNOW BEST

Thelma Brenner, an elegant woman raised in Boston, was always dieting. She ate lots of peanuts at meals in an attempt to shed some weight. I asked Marie, "Why peanuts, a high-fat, salty snack, to lose weight?" Marie said, "That's Thelma." Marie's mother was not in any way what one would term excessively overweight. She struggled with the same ten to fifteen pounds that Marie does. (In the last stages of cancer, Thelma actually called a good friend and said, "Harriet, I'm finally thin. You should see my waist.") According to Marie, "Mother defined 'fat' as anyone weighing over 135 pounds."

IS YOUR EARLY PROGRAMMING PLAYING A STARRING ROLE?

Marie and I frequently talk about how her mother's early programming has continued to play a starring role in her desire to lose weight and simultaneously prevented her from accomplishing her goal. In addition to constant dieting in front of Marie (more on this later in the chapter), Thelma made comments to her as a child when she brought home clothes for her to try on. She would look Marie over, tilt her head, and say with a lilt, "That's not so bad." In her twenties, when Marie would weigh herself and the scale would indicate 140 pounds, Thelma would say once again, with the same expression and cadence, "That's not so bad." Throughout her life, Thelma would critique Marie's outfits. She would look Marie up and down, pause, inhale, and remark, "That's not your *best* look." (Marie and *her* daughter now use that same expression in good-hearted jest when they try on clothes together. No compulsive repetition applies— Marie stopped the pattern.)

WHAT'S KEPT *YOU* FROM FLIPPING?

Thelma read Adele Davis's *Let's Eat Right to Keep Fit* (my own mother had this book) at the dinner table and kept a small pad of paper at her side during all meals to jot down her calories. (She got the idea from Pamela Harriman, ambassador to France, who used to keep a pad at her side to mark the mistakes made by her staff.) She insisted that Marie drink the "meat juice" (think of the fat and calories!) for the B vitamins. Marie admits she doesn't know where Thelma got that idea.

ANYONE FOR A TALL GLASS OF MEAT JUICE?

Marie was on a cocktail of rainbow diet pills at sixteen, and when she did finally hit 135 pounds, Thelma said, with a smile, "Well, now, let's try for 125." The message to Marie was, you'll *never* be thin enough. Finally, Thelma would frequently point out other women and indicate to Marie, "Now *she* has the figure for that outfit." These comments, though by no means meant to intentionally harm, became Marie's mental graffiti.

It became immediately apparent to me that in order for Marie to successfully flip she had to reclaim her "metabolism." Basically, she needed to flip the phrase "That's not so bad" into "That's pretty good" and ultimately get to "Hey, that's *very* good!" Marie's mental graffiti needed some editing. How did she do it, and how can you do it? First, she talked about it. Just the process of actively talking about her mom, her early impression of her own body, and her current feeling about her body (and agreeing to let me talk about it in this book) was extremely helpful. I urge you, as I did in Chapter 1, to do the same. Start talking about your early programming.

EDIT YOUR MENTAL GRAFFITI

Was It More About Her Than You?

Examine the programming. I realize that it is very difficult to do this in an objective, detached manner, but ultimately that is what's required. Try to gain an insight into your mother's motivation. Was it more about her than you? Why was Thelma so committed to Marie's thinness? Was it for Marie's benefit, as she clearly believed that Marie would be happier thin, or was it about Thelma's not wanting a non-thin daughter, which would have been a reflection on her as a parent. Review the context of your mother's life at the time she was programming you. It's much easier to do this as an adult than when you were a child. Were your parents in a happy relationship? What opportunities as a young woman did your mother have apart from parenting? What relationship did she have with her own parents? By thinking about these and other factors, you may gain an insight into what motivated your mother to expose you to this sort of programming. Please realize that none of this necessarily indicates that your mother didn't love you (Thelma loved Marie). Thelma, too, was a product of conditioning. Once you gain an understanding of your mother's frustration and motivation, you can begin to apply a commonsense approach to your feelings in this area.

REVIEW THE CONTEXT OF YOUR MOTHER'S LIFE

Once you see that none of this programming has any basis in truth, you can begin the deprogramming process. You will understand that *you* and *only you* control your metabolism. Who literally puts food in your mouth? You do. Who actually does the exercising? You do. Just telling Marie to "eat less, exercise more" is worthless advice without getting to the core of her problem. This is essentially the process Marie went through to overcome her early programming.

The challenge is for her to stop believing when she looks in the mirror that she's "not so bad."

To date, Marie is down approximately fifteen pounds. She is following my exercise prescription and performing more strength and resistance exercise than she has in the past. Previously, Marie was following a plan heavily dominated by cardiovascular exercise. You can readily see the difference in her body's composition and especially in her arms. They look great. We are striving for her to eat 1,200 calories a day consisting of vegetables, fruits, and lean protein to lose the last few pounds. Marie and I are both "in process." Are we cured? Are we thin for life? Are we flipped for life? I strongly believe so, but it is a never-ending process. Even with a successful career, a family, a beautiful home, and a great group of friends, Marie continues to do battle with her "mother as her metabolism." But today, Marie is winning.

Dieting Moms

Like Thelma Brenner, some mothers place too much pressure on themselves to be thin, and this behavior then affects their daughters' attitudes toward food, dieting, and body image. Ira Sacker, M.D., coauthor of the book *Dying to Be Thin*, states, "Some of my patients, who are just out of nursery school, tell me that they're fat. Turns out that their moms are saying the same thing about themselves." Innocently, your mother's behavior may have made an imprint on you very early in life. Think back and recall if that's the case. If so, how have you related to it over the years? Has it hampered your weight-loss goals?

Regardless of whether your mother consciously or subconsciously placed undue emphasis on diet, weight, and body image, this programming prompts you to value yourself according to these issues. From a very early age, as early as nursery school, women start to develop the mental graffiti that makes little sense but manages to grow and supplant all reason. This mental graffiti includes thoughts such as "I'll never be thin enough," "Who would ever want me? I'm ugly, unattractive and fat," and "I just can't lose weight. Why even try?" These play over and over again in your head and totally thwart your desire to succeed at weight loss. It can drive a woman of any age to distraction and irrational behavior.

YOU SHOULD SEE
HER ARMS

WHAT'S
KEPT *YOU*
FROM
FLIPPING?

248

WOMEN START TO
DEVELOP MENTAL
GRAFFITI EARLY ON

Here are a few examples of ways in which this unfortunate programming affects some women. Sane adult women will starve themselves before seeing their aging mothers. This frequently occurs before a holiday or some big family event, such as a wedding. First, the daughter generally binges on food just from thinking about having to see her mother. Then, a few weeks before the event, the daughter is exercising around the clock, starving, and generally making everyone around her (including her personal trainer) crazy. There is an exaggerated fear of rejection. Many of these women have successful careers, marriages, relationships with their own children, and friendships—you name it (think Marie). But once their mothers (or just the thought of their mothers) enter the picture, everything changes and they are once again unhappy children desperately seeking the approval of their mothers. That approval, they believe, will only come from reducing their body weight. Are you following a similar pattern?

ARE YOU STILL SEEKING APPROVAL FROM YOUR MOTHER?

Ask yourself, "Is my mother my metabolism? Does my mother, whether alive or not, continue to influence my relationship with *my* body image and *my* weight?" I know for a fact that some women remain overweight as a way of getting back at their mothers. Some strongly disliked the constant emphasis their mothers (or fathers) placed on physical appearance and body weight above any other accomplishment. Many have shared the stories of daily weigh-ins, forced diets, and "fat camps." Some were told that they could *not* go to the country club at that weight. Therefore, by staying overweight, the daughter now feels she is prevailing and the one in control. Mind you, in many instances, the mother is no longer alive.

Don't Fulfill the "Negative" Prophecy

Unfortunately, some women, consciously or subconsciously, are fulfilling their mothers' "failure" prophecy. A mother led her daughter to believe that she ultimately would be a failure at weight loss, so she simply became one. She reinforced the "negative" prophecy. Think about it. Do you ever say or think to yourself, "Well, Mom, you always said I was a fat loser? Look at me now. I did it!" Unfortunately, you know and I know that by staying overweight you are only hurting one person—yourself. Think about that for a moment. By stay-

WHO DO YOU REALLY HURT BY BEING OVERWEIGHT?

I have often seen these patterns apply to each female family member. I touched upon this earlier in Chapter 6, when I cited the excuse "My sisters and I are all overweight, so it must be our genes." No, my experience is that all of you have weight issues, perhaps provoked by an overly strict mother or father, a permissive parent who praised with food, or a mother who constantly dieted and discussed body weight. You need to explore your behavior. All overweight individuals need to explore their first relationship with food, body image, and weight rather than blame their genes.

ing overweight, by refusing to flip, the only person you hurt is you. If you flip, you are the winner, not your mother!

Fathers and Daughters

In October 2001, new research presented by the North American Association for the Study of Obesity indicated that "parents, especially fathers, have considerable influence in promoting healthy lifestyles for their daughters." They actually found that a daughter's activity patterns are most likely to be affected by her father's activity patterns. This is important for every father to know. Your commitment to activity and exercise has a strong influence on how your daughter will embrace activity and exercise. The women reading this book should stop for a moment and think about their fathers' activity pattern. Did Dad jog, play tennis, lift weights, or swim? Maybe he golfed, skied, or took long bike rides with you when you were growing up. Think about it and how this may have affected you.

LIKE FATHER
LIKE DAUGHTER?

Unfortunately, many women were raised at a time when girls were not encouraged to play sports by either their mothers or their fathers. We know now that participating in sports can have an overwhelmingly positive influence on young women with regard to self-esteem, physical ability, and the opportunity to learn to be a team player. By observing an active father, a daughter may be more likely to duplicate that behavior.

Be a Healthy Role Model

For years, I have been cautioned by clients and friends, some of whom are psychologists or psychiatrists, that I should never place undue emphasis on body weight and appearance in front of my children, especially my daughter, given the fact that I am in this business. As I said in the first chapter, I am very aware of the potential negative impact this could create. Many women who suffer from anorexia and bulimia were reared by lean fathers who were overly critical when it came to appearance and body weight. I never mention weight to my daughter—or to anyone else's children, for that matter. I don't even tell kids, mine included, that I am in the weight-loss business. I want to be a good role model, making healthy food choices and regularly exercising, but I don't make it an issue. Rather, I want kids to view exercise and healthy eating as a way of life, just like going to work, playing, and watching television. I exercise, as does my wife, anywhere from three to four times a week.

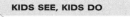

KIDS SEE, KIDS DO

We also make activity with the kids fun, whether it be swimming every Sunday in our building's pool, playing at the beach across the street from our home, or running to my office. We make it fun. We make it a part of life. I know you can do the same. It's actually quite easy to incorporate activity into your family's routine. It doesn't cost very much, nor does it take much time. Kids just want to be with their parents. And don't forget the cliché "Monkey see, monkey do"—"Kids see, kids do."

Women in Love

A woman is single, and she is trying to get on the dating circuit. She is exercising, dieting, dating, exercising, dieting, dating, and spending the majority of her time with other women who are doing the same. Then she meets someone. She goes out to dinner with "him" more and more frequently. This guy likes to eat. He likes to drink. He resents the time she devotes on weekend mornings to exercise. Gradually she starts to gain some weight. But hey, she's in love. Someone loves her, so she's okay with a few extra inches here and a few additional pounds there. Sure, her friends notice a subtle change, but they don't have a boyfriend or a husband so perhaps they are jealous—maybe they are even glad that she gained some weight. Does this sound like you or someone you know?

My weight-loss management firm, Jim Karas Personal Training,

LLC, had a client we'll call Jane. She had nursed her husband through a long illness. Not long after he died, she called my office to begin a program to lose the thirty-five additional pounds she had gained. Jane was ready to flip. For the next nine months, Jane was a model client. She lost almost thirty pounds and told us she felt and looked the best she had in years.

Then Jane met "Dick." Almost from their first date, she started to gain weight. Dick liked steak. Dick liked Mexican food. Dick was so much "fun." When one of my staff asked Jane why she was eating all of these high-calorie foods, she said, "I have to. He likes to share entrées and this is the food he likes." Jane was in her fifties but still allowing someone to dictate what she put in her mouth. When I called her to talk about her weight gain, Jane rushed me off the phone and told me she would call back the next day. She never did.

Then Jane started to skip her exercise sessions, something she had never done before, and ultimately left a message on our office voice mail telling us that Dick didn't want her to train with us anymore. I called her more than a dozen times over the next two weeks. I use all the tricks when people are avoiding me: I block the caller ID (so they don't know it's me calling) and I phone in the morning, at dinner-time, or around 10:00 A.M. on a Sunday. Jane was never in, and we didn't hear from her again.

Do men stop playing golf for a relationship? Do men quit their weekly card game? Do men enjoy Lean Cuisine or cottage cheese and pineapple for dinner? Okay, maybe some do, but not the majority. No, even today, many women will put the needs of a man ahead of their own. He comes first. Don't get angry with me for saying these things, but ask yourself: "Should a man be threatened by my desire to maintain good health and a lean body weight?" Absolutely not, if he's the right man!

If this relationship works, it may turn into a marriage, which may result in children, more financial success, more eating out, more travel, more buffets, more celebratory dinners. Do you see where I am headed? What will you weigh at the end of all this? Yes, fall in love. Yes, enjoy the person you are with. Share common interests. But don't let a relationship curtail your flip. This does not have to happen.

Women and Families

I touched on making time for the right food choices in Chapter 3, "'I Don't Have the Time,'" but I feel it requires a little more attention. Back in your "single" days, the only person (at least for most young women) you had to worry about feeding was you. You munched on salads, had nothing but "your kind of food" in the refrigerator, and were always about to start or stop another "lose weight fast" drastic diet. Your weight stayed under control. Then you got married. Okay, now you have two to worry about. After a while, along come the kids. Now you are shopping and cooking for three, four, five, or more. Mealtimes can be a challenge. The kids want macaroni and cheese, your husband wants pizza, and you want to flip and eat grilled chicken with steamed broccoli. Do you serve three different meals? Of course not. Who has time to do that? So, whose needs get pushed aside? Most likely, yours. You end up picking around the macaroni or deluding yourself into believing that the crust of the pizza is not so bad.

Do Yourself a Favor

Put yourself first. If your husband and kids don't like grilled chicken with broccoli, then point to the refrigerator and tell them that smoked turkey is in there if they would like to make a sandwich. Or alternate dinners. One night, make their macaroni and cheese (while you flip and enjoy "your kind of food"), the next night make whatever you want.

On weekends, especially, make enough so that there will be leftovers. You have more time. Buy a couple of pounds of boneless, skin-

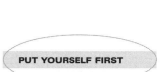

PUT YOURSELF FIRST

WHEN YOU FLIP, THE WHOLE FAMILY BENEFITS

The more you integrate healthier food into *your* diet, the more your whole family benefits. If your kids and spouse see you eating certain foods, or start to try other foods because you are preparing them, they will soon acquire a taste for them. Or don't even tell them. Just change to a lower calorie salad dressing, or go from full-fat mayo to "light." Don't make it a big issue, and I bet your family won't even notice.

less chicken breast or a fresh turkey breast. On Sunday, grill the chicken (and grill whatever your kids want at the same time) or cook the turkey breast. Then, place your food in containers so that you have meals for the first few days of the week. You can prepare whatever the family wants knowing that your food is ready to go.

In the *Flip the Switch* Seven-Day Jump-Start Eating Plan (pages 123–124), I included products to make meals easy. I don't want you to think mealtime has to be difficult and time-consuming. I just want you to be able to cook for your family and stay on the plan. Plan, plan, plan, and it works.

Women and Aging

We all age. There simply is no way around it, but the psychological experience can be more difficult for women than for men. Society evolves, technology improves, and a woman may someday be president—but if she is, the media will discuss her hair and clothing much more so than a male candidate's, if his is even discussed. Women still tend to be judged more by their appearance than are men. For many women, appearance is power. As a woman ages, she may feel her power begin to wane. Of course, this is a ridiculous notion. But women diet more than men, exercise more than men, and have more plastic surgery than men (though men are gaining on them), all in an effort to fight the aging process. The fact is, men are evaluated less by their appearance and thus aging is less apt to hamper their careers or affect them emotionally. But age, as you'll see in Chapter 10, " 'It's Just Too Late,' " shouldn't stop you from flipping. In fact, you'll soon realize that flipping is one of the best steps you can take to age with grace, confidence, and strength. Every woman deserves that.

What's a Woman to Do?

As I discussed at the beginning of this chapter, it is harder for women to keep their body weight down because of their size, percent of body fat, menstruation, childbearing, and menopause. Add to this anxiety or depression, which tends to affect more women than men, and you can readily see how weight loss is tougher for women. So what are you to do?

First, you must realize that this situation is totally manageable. I have coached many women of all ages to successful weight loss. Now, this requires dedication and discipline. This is serious work. But it is a path that ultimately will lead any woman to feel strong, sexy, and capable of conquering almost anything. You'll believe that you can "get your body back." And, like many of my female clients, you may end up with a better body than you had in the first place!

Obsessive Behavior or Intelligent Behavior?

Often when I meet a woman and tell her what profession I am in, she will launch into a thirty-minute diatribe on her "neighbor" who is obsessed with eating and exercise: "My neighbor is always carrying water with her. She looks ridiculous." I think drinking water is smart. If carrying it with you (I do!) helps you to get it down, what's the problem? Then the woman says, "My neighbor is always ordering everything on the side. [I do!] Salad dressing on the side and sauce on the side. It's embarrassing to be out with her." I think ordering everything on the side is the smartest, simplest thing you can do (remember, I told you to do it in Chapter 7). As I've said before, it can knock off hundreds if not thousands of calories from your eating plan. Finally, the woman says, "And what is with all this exercise? I am so sick of her rushing off to the gym. She is just obsessed with all this." I totally disagree. To me, this neighbor sounds smart. She is following through with a plan and succeeding at weight loss. Is the woman criticizing her neighbor winning her battle with the scale? I'll let you decide.

Just to clarify, the neighbor is not one of those poor souls I talked about earlier who run past your window day and night, night and day. This is someone who carves out the time to perform strength and resistance exercise and follows through with an intelligent, low-calorie eating plan.

Plastic Surgery

If you feel you need plastic surgery, then have it. But please do yourself a big favor. Before you touch anything, from your face to your eyes to your breasts to your thighs, you must first lose any unwanted

O, The Oprah Magazine, ran a great piece by Lise Funderberg on my program featuring my client Diane Sawyer. In this article, Diane said that losing twenty-five pounds, changing her body's composition, and feeling strong helped her get her "it" back. Many women who saw the piece commented on that one line. Here we have a woman in her mid-fifties, one of television's most successful journalists, happily married to a very accomplished man, with beautiful homes, great friends, the whole shebang—what any observer would consider an "ideal" life—and still she was coping with the whole issue of body image, body weight, and aging. Succeeding at weight loss, she felt she got her "it" back. Of course, we never knew that she'd lost her "it," but she did. Diane's coming forth and being honest about that feeling was inspirational to many women. They told me so in e-mails, phone calls, and letters. Don't think that stars and celebrities are immune; they aren't. They struggle with these issues just as much as you do. The only difference is that they have to do it with millions of people watching their every move. Talk about pressure.

LOSE THE WEIGHT
BEFORE YOU NIP
AND TUCK

weight. I am enraged when I hear from a client that a plastic surgeon said, "First do the face. That will motivate you to lose the weight." Wrong, wrong, wrong. You must be at optimal body weight before you have any type of cosmetic procedure. You should have "work done" on your face or your body when it is in proper proportion and at a desirable weight, or else the results will be disappointing (and in some cases disastrous). Never have liposuction done unless you are at your optimal weight and plan on staying there for the rest of your life. I have heard countless women tell me that after they had lipo on their thighs, they began gaining weight in the abdominal area and in their behind. And furthermore, contrary to popular belief, liposuction is for fine-tuning. It should *never* be used to eliminate a dramatic amount of weight or fat.

One final point: Plastic surgery is surgery. There are risks. Also, realize that cosmetic surgery does not address interior issues. Only you can do that.

"Just Accept It"

I can't tell you how much I disagree with this message. By "just accepting" being overweight as a function of aging, a woman is increasing her risk of everything from heart disease and cancer to joint

> ### BYPASS IT: GASTRIC, THAT IS
>
> Gastric bypass procedures are complicated and dangerous. This surgery results in an abnormally small stomach, forcing you to eat very small portions of food for the rest of your life. There is no turning back. Why not skip the surgery and just eat the small portions? Why are you putting your life in jeopardy by having major elective surgery? This is really a last resort for seriously obese individuals who emotionally can't get control of their weight or whose doctors may decide that such a procedure is necessary to save their lives.

replacements and loss of independence. The next chapter, "'It's Just Too Late,'" explores many of the issues surrounding successful aging and body weight. Never accept being overweight as a function of age or gender. Make the decision to fight it and be victorious.

GAINING WEIGHT IS NOT A FUNCTION OF AGING

Having It All

There is one more point about women and body weight. Some women cannot accept "having it all." There is a fear that they cannot, or should not, have a career, a relationship, children, family, friends, *and* a lean body. I have heard this remark many times, and to this day am still shocked by it. A woman ages and becomes more confident and successful, but to balance things out, she moves up in body weight. It's almost a form of self-punishment. This increase in weight then overshadows all of her other accomplishments. Men rarely embrace such thinking.

WHY NOT HAVE IT ALL?

The Heart of the Matter

Let me leave you with a startling statistic. As I am finishing this chapter with the television on in the background, I hear Oprah report on her show that "one out of every two women will die of heart disease. It kills approximately half a million women a year." This same statistic was also reported in the *New York Times*. Think about that: One out of two women will die of heart disease. In surveys, most women fear breast cancer far more than heart disease, though its mortality rate is, in fact, lower. (About 40,200 women die of breast cancer annually.) In addition, the *New York Times* reported that "women are more likely than men to die within a year of having a heart attack, or to have a second heart attack during the six years after the first one. Similarly, women do not fare as well as men after bypass surgery or other procedures that are used to open blocked coronary arteries." The reason for this is not clear, although it is noted that most women have other conditions, such as diabetes or stroke, in addition to the heart disease that color their prognosis.

Does that motivate you to flip?

You Control Your Body

Despite all these factors—mothers, fathers, societal pressure, aging, and plain old biology—I urge you, as I have from the beginning, to believe in the fact that *you control your body*. It's your body. No one else can make you eat; no one else can keep you from exercising.

PUTTING IT ALL TOGETHER TO FLIP

- Weight loss is more difficult for women than men, but it's by no means impossible.

- Biology alone does not determine destiny—you do.

- To achieve successful weight loss, women must understand the six physiological factors that affect the Balance of Energy Equation.

- Edit or eliminate negative mental graffiti and replace it with positive mental graffiti. Turn *can't* into *can*.

- Explore your relationships with your mother, father, and siblings.

- Life consists of choices: Choose to be a success at weight loss.

10 "It's Just Too Late"

My firm, Jim Karas Personal Training, LLC, has many clients who are in their seventies, eighties, and even nineties. Most of them come to my firm as a result of a personal referral. "Mrs. Smith," a seventy-five-year-old client, has lunch with her friend "Mrs. Jones," whom she hasn't seen for several months. Upon seeing a thinner Mrs. Smith stride to the table full of confidence, with great color in her skin and her shoulders back, Mrs. Jones exclaims, "You look great! Have you had something done? I can't put my finger on it, but I haven't seen you look this good in years. What is your secret?" Mrs. Smith replies, "I have a personal fitness trainer who comes to my home three times a week to work out with me. He has helped me with my stamina and posture, my bone density is up, I've lost twelve pounds, and I feel energized." Mrs. Jones replies, "Please, can I have his number?"

You can flip at any age and achieve significant mental and physical benefits. According to the *Mayo Clinic's Guide to Successful Aging,* "genes account for only about one third of the effects of aging; the rest are due mainly to lifestyle and environment." Does this surprise you? You may have been under the impression that it was all predetermined by your genes. This is not the case. How you age is basically determined by you. This chapter begins by exploring the various ways in which the human body physically ages.

Can the Aging Process Be Slowed?

A Tufts University case study conclusively proved that individuals in their nineties who performed strength and resistance exercises three times a week for eight weeks increased their strength by 300 percent. Ponder for just a moment what a 300 percent increase in strength can contribute to both the body and the mind. In only eight weeks of con-

> "AGE IS OF NO IMPORTANCE UNLESS YOU ARE CHEESE."
> —BILLIE BURKE

sistent strength and resistance exercise, people in their nineties increased their strength 300 percent! Consider the effects after eight more weeks, or six months, or one year! Much of what we have considered "normal" about aging has little or nothing to do with the physical process of aging. What we have witnessed instead is a lack of muscle use, which leads to muscular atrophy. This degenerative process is termed sarcopenia. As we have learned, muscular atrophy leads to a reduced metabolism and excess body weight, which in turn creates a number of negative effects for the human body, such as diabetes, heart disease, and cancer.

I want you to reread the anecdote at the beginning of this chapter to underscore the benefits that strength and resistance exercise produced for "Mrs. Smith." Despite dramatic success stories such as hers, I still encounter resistance from older individuals, especially women, who have sought my assistance. They make comments such as, "All this exercise is just not for me. My daughter and son-in-law are always trying to get me to do it and I just don't want to. And furthermore, I'm not going to let one of those trainers beat me up and injure me." At one new client meeting, a woman in her late seventies kept repeating, "I don't want to be injured, I don't want to be sore." Each time she expressed this concern, I would attempt to allay her fears by saying, "That's not how we treat our clients. We start slowly, establish what you feel comfortable doing, then systematically progress your plan. We never injure our clients." My reassurances still did not dispel her fear. Finally, I asked, "Who has put this notion into your head that we are going to injure you?" She replied, "No one. I am just really frightened to give this a try. I feel it's just too late."

Take the Fear Out of Exercise

I have to admit that I understand why older people make this type of remark. Most individuals, especially those over sixty, have never performed strength and resistance exercises. It all just seems so foreign. It simply wasn't done when they were younger. Some played tennis or golf, and that was considered being "active." Plus, many of us have seen unprofessional fitness trainers depicted on television, in films, in infomercials or advertisements who yell at their clients and behave like drill sergeants. They scream, "one more, come on, go for the burn," or something along those lines. No one at any age appreciates this approach. Berating does not motivate; positive reinforcement does.

Why Act Your Age?

When someone sees all the positive effects of intelligent exercise sitting in front of him or her, then the decision is infinitely easier to make, as it was for Mrs. Jones in the opening anecdote. Wouldn't you want to look better, feel better, minimize pain, stand straighter, and have more energy, especially as you are getting older? In our society, older individuals are often told, "Act your age," but this dictate frequently strips them of their minds, mobility, and independent lifestyles, and can lead to depression. Observe the elderly. Think about your Aunt Sophie or Uncle Harry. Do they socialize, surf the Internet, dance, travel, and perform strength and resistance exercise? Or do they watch television (predominantly reruns of *Murder She Wrote* and *Matlock*), sleep, regale you with their most recent illness, and shuffle through a round of nine holes of golf once a week? Which behavior pattern represents acting his or her age? What is eighty supposed to seem like? That is up to you. The words *vibrant, full of energy, alert,* and *curious* should be used to describe an individual at any age. Those who flip the switch by watching their diet and weight and by incorporating strength and resistance exercise into their lives shave years off of their appearance, drastically improve their energy level, dramatically slow the aging process, and continue living rich, independent lives.

It's Never Too Late to Flip

Take a look around you—who's going to the gym? According to the *New York Times,* "Americans older

---

AGING WELL

In his book *Aging Well,* Harvard Medical School psychiatrist George Vaillant has an impressive take on the subject. He states that the most important psychological predictor of aging well is learning how "to cope: to sublimate, rechannel, diffuse and dispense with envy, anger, aggression and revenge. No stewing. No dwelling." After reading this, I stopped and thought for a moment. Most of the people I know in their seventies (my mother-in-law and father-in law included), eighties, and nineties who appear so happy and content are doing just that.

than 55 are the fastest-growing segment of the health club market and visit the gym more often—an average of 97 days a year—than any other age group. But that's only about 7.3 million people out of the 59 million Americans over 55. One in three Americans is sedentary. There's a huge percentage of the public for whom good nutrition and exercise hasn't even appeared on the radar screen."

As the Tufts University research indicates, as one ages, the results produced by strength and resistance exercise are dramatic. Further research shows that in addition to building lean muscle tissue and boosting metabolism, the whole process of flipping produces the following benefits.

It Strengthens Your Heart

Barry Franklin, Ph.D., director of the cardiac rehabilitation program at William Beaumont Hospital in Royal Oak, Michigan, says, "Don't underestimate the heart benefits of weight training." In fact, the American Heart Association now recommends resistance training to prevent and treat heart disease:

- Resistance training makes the heart more efficient. In the past, only cardiovascular exercise was thought to make the heart more efficient. Now, it has been proved that strength and resistance exercise also gets the job done.

- Weight training can lower your resting heart rate and blood pressure. Once again, in the past, physicians and researchers believed only cardio could accomplish these goals. Now it is proved that strength and resistance exercise produces the same results.

- The stronger your muscles are, the less strain you place on your heart when you do something physical. Consider all the daily activities you perform, such as carrying groceries, cleaning the house, and taking out the trash, all of which require physical exertion. These and so many more tasks are made easier by building stronger muscles.

Why perform only cardiovascular exercise to strengthen your heart and burn a few additional calories when you can perform strength and resistance exercise that strengthens your heart, builds lean muscle tissue, lowers your blood pressure, places less strain on your heart, and burns additional calories twenty-four hours a day, seven days a week, 365 days a year?

It Reduces Hypertension

Recently, it was reported that "middle-age risk of hypertension is staggeringly high. A study predicts that nine out of ten middle-aged Americans will, at some point, develop high blood pressure, a disorder called the silent killer because it insidiously increases the risk of heart attack and stroke." Strength and resistance exercise and weight loss both contribute to a reduction in high blood pressure. To complement your strength and resistance exercises, the *Flip the Switch* Jump-Start Seven-Day Eating Plan and the eating rules I urge you to follow are very high in fruits and vegetables, which are packed with antioxidants and contribute to your blood vessels remaining elastic and your heart beating strongly. When you flip, you look better, feel better, and significantly reduce your risk of heart disease. Remember the statistic I cited at the end of the previous chapter: One out of every two women will die of heart disease. This is not what I want for any of you.

FIGHT HIGH BLOOD
PRESSURE WITH THE FLIP

It Strengthens Your Bones

When you perform strength and resistance exercise, we've established that you place stress on your muscles. But in addition to stressing the muscles, strength and resistance exercise also stresses the bones that are attached to those muscles. (Don't be frightened by the word *stresses*—this is good stress, not bad.) In the previous chapter, I discussed how bone is an "active" tissue continually going through the process of losing and replacing itself. This process is termed "remodeling." Strength and resistance exercises stimulate the bone-building cells to respond and perform their job more regularly and effectively. Therefore, as a net effect, strength and resistance exercise can slow, if not stall, bone loss throughout the body. This is especially important as we age. Here are some recent findings:

Why Build Bone?

- *Newsweek:* "Twenty-four percent of people over 50 who suffer a hip fracture die within the year."

- The Mayo Clinic: "One out of six women will fracture a hip during their lifetime and up to twenty-five percent of all people in nursing homes are there as a result of a hip fracture."

- Rheumatic Diseases Clinics of North America: "Almost 30 percent of all hip fractures occur in men."

Long known as a problem affecting women past menopause, osteoporosis is now emerging as a problem among older men as well. Fewer men than women do break a hip, but there's a steep increase in the number of fractures in men after age seventy-five. Flipping is not an

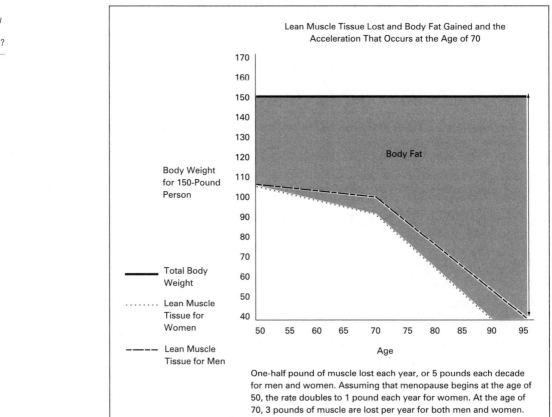

Lean Muscle Tissue Lost and Body Fat Gained and the Acceleration That Occurs at the Age of 70

Body Fat

Body Weight for 150-Pound Person

——— Total Body Weight

.... Lean Muscle Tissue for Women

– – – Lean Muscle Tissue for Men

Age

One-half pound of muscle lost each year, or 5 pounds each decade for men and women. Assuming that menopause begins at the age of 50, the rate doubles to 1 pound each year for women. At the age of 70, 3 pounds of muscle are lost per year for both men and women.

option for many of the elderly with osteoporosis. On the contrary, it is a necessity.

It Stops the Decline in Lean Muscle Tissue

Studies continue to indicate that regular strength and resistance exercise can deter what was once thought to be an inevitable decline in muscle mass. In fact, a three-year study published in September 2001 in the *Journal of the American Medical Association* showed that older and younger healthy men create new muscle proteins at similar rates. Similar rates! What does this tell us? Obviously, regardless of one's age, new muscle proteins (the building blocks for muscle development) can be created at any time in life and the aging process dramatically slowed.

Additionally, we have long observed that as individuals age, they not only experience a reduction in their muscle mass but also lose a large percentage of the "fast twitch" muscle fibers. These fast-twitch muscle fibers are associated with our ability to quickly respond to a change in our physical environment. We trip or slip and these fast-twitch muscle fibers react to that change. Their reaction, in part, helps us to avoid falls. A team of researchers at Ball State University in Muncie, Indiana, recently concluded that strength and resistance exercise significantly improves an individual's fast-twitch muscle

YOU CAN GROW LEAN MUSCLE TISSUE AT ANY AGE

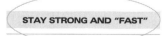

STAY STRONG AND "FAST"

fibers and at the same time rejuvenates them. Fewer falls or no falls mean a more independent lifestyle for all Americans, especially older Americans.

It Helps You Maintain Independence

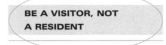
BE A VISITOR, NOT
A RESIDENT

Remember what I said earlier about all the daily activities you perform, such as carrying groceries, cleaning the house, and taking out the trash? All of these tasks and so many more are made easier by building stronger muscles. Plus, according to the *Wall Street Journal,* stronger muscles "let [the elderly] stay independent and out of the nursing home into advanced old age."

I want to revisit Chapter 1 for a moment. Do you recall my discussion of the fear factor to motivate the flip? I discussed a client who had had a heart attack and flipped for a brief period of time out of fear; unfortunately, he flipped back when his fear dissipated. The same fear factor is a powerful motivator to convince older individuals that they can continue their independent lifestyles by flipping. I have received numerous phone calls from people who have said, "My close friend just fell and broke her hip. Now she is in a nursing home and I can barely stand to visit her. It is so depressing in there. What can I do to prevent this from happening to me?" These individuals generally listen to everything my staff or I have to say. Many have *never* exercised or watched their caloric intake in their entire lives. Yet, they flip and stay flipped because they do not want to end up in a nursing home or some other assisted-living facility.

It Works at Any Age

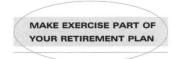
MAKE EXERCISE PART OF
YOUR RETIREMENT PLAN

According to Dr. Benjamin Levine, associate professor of internal medicine and director of the Institute for Exercise and Environmental Medicine, "starting an exercise program when older is still useful and can combat the effects of aging. . . . Moreover, if you *stop* exercise, you can lose what you have gained relatively quickly. Therefore, exercise must be a lifelong health habit—like brushing your teeth and taking a shower—that can and should be sustained throughout life."

If you want to live independently, in your home, for the rest of your life, there is only one answer to being physically and mentally able to achieve that goal—you must flip the switch *now*. Maybe you don't feel old at the moment, but you've heard that "life is short." I recently read an interview with former President Bill Clinton in which he was asked if he felt old at fifty-five years of age. "No, but it doesn't seem so long ago that I was twenty," he remarked. Time does move rapidly. So, if you aren't elderly now, it's coming sooner than you think. Plan for your *body's* retirement just as you are urged to plan for other aspects of your retirement such as housing, finances, and health care.

It Chases the Blues Away—Come On, Get Happy

Depression affects between 25 and 30 percent of all individuals after the age of sixty. Many times, it goes undiagnosed. "Exercise, whether in the form of strength training, stretching or walking, can provide a much needed emotional boost to frail elderly men and women," according to researchers from the Washington University School of Medicine in St. Louis. These researchers discovered that participants experienced a marked improvement in overall emotional health and, specifically, in how they felt about themselves. We also know that exercise appears to relieve anxiety, stress, low self-esteem, and sleeplessness. Flipping can be just the answer to shaking the blues. In addition to the exercise, in particular strength and resistance training, certain foods such as fruits and vegetables, which are packed with antioxidants, can enhance mood.

Researchers from Emory University School of Medicine in Atlanta found that depressed people age sixty and older with hypertension developed heart failure at more than double the rate of those who were not depressed. As I previously indicated, nine out of ten individuals will suffer from hypertension. Hypertension places additional stress on the heart. The researchers found that depression also causes excessive stimulation of the body's nervous system, which controls heart rate and breathing. Therefore, between the high blood pressure and the depression, you are taxing your heart and placing yourself at a high risk for heart disease. Flipping can reverse both of these negative forces.

Though women in general suffer more frequently from depression, they also are more likely to seek treatment. Men are ten times more likely to commit suicide after the age of eighty-five. It is widely

FLIPPING GIVES YOU AN EMOTIONAL BOOST

HIGH BLOOD PRESSURE AND DEPRESSION = INCREASED RISK OF HEART FAILURE believed that as the baby boomers age, this difference will be less dramatic, since many men of that generation are more accustomed to seeking psychological help. But in the meantime, keep an eye on your father, grandfather, or older male friend and watch for the warning signs of depression. If you see any, encourage them to flip.

Finally, in Chapters 3 and 8 we discussed which exercise time and place options are best for you. Specifically for seniors, I like the health club/gym option because of the social aspect. Numerous studies show that the more socially active an individual remains, the less apt he or she is to experience bouts of depression.

It Helps You Say "So Long" to Pain

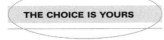

A client and I were recently having lunch. For years, her mother has struggled with her weight and now, in her early eighties, she has terrible arthritis in both knees. *Three* doctors told her she would be in a wheelchair within a year. Upon hearing this, my client took over. She said, "Mother, the choice is yours. Either you start watching what you eat, exercise, and lose weight, or you're in the chair. I will do anything, I mean anything, to help you succeed, but if you decide to opt for the chair, you can count me out." Well, her mother flipped and is down twenty-two pounds (she still has more to go) and is virtually pain-free. Remember, three doctors predicted she would end up in a wheelchair. Not one recommended that she flip and make a commitment to lose weight and exercise.

I have one more point to make about excessive cardiovascular exercise, which I discussed in Chapter 8, and staying pain-free. Remember the cardio fanatics running by your window every hour? These individuals are accelerating the deterioration of their joints. The body's joints were not designed to withstand the pounding and jarring repetition of running. If you are one of these individuals, then consider cutting back. If you have friends or family members whose behavior is similar, talk with them about cutting back on all this excessive cardio and urge them to embrace strength and resistance exercise. Not only will they reap the rewards of building lean muscle tissue, boosting their metabolism, improving their posture, and enhancing their body composition, they will reduce if not eliminate the risk of joint-related pain. Also, mention to them that many case

AGING JOINTS DON'T
LIKE POUNDING

WHAT IS ARTHRITIS?

As the body ages, arthritis, a diminishing of the body's cartilage, takes place. Cartilage is like a washer in between a nut and a bolt. Without the washer, the nut and the bolt would grind together. That is what happens when you lose cartilage. The bone grating on bone will progressively cause inflammation, pain, and discomfort. The degree to which arthritis affects the body depends upon a number of variables, which include genetics, gender, activity, body weight, and alignment. It is widely believed that a reduction in body weight will undoubtedly diminish some if not all of the pain of arthritis. In addition, performing strength and resistance exercise will help to strengthen the tendons, ligaments, and muscles that surround the joint. That reinforcement will take pressure off and subsequently alleviate pain in the weakened area. Water is used to lubricate cartilage in the body, so staying well hydrated by drinking water and eating high-water-content foods will also minimize the pain.

studies show that exercise for less than an hour each day can enhance immunity, and exercise for more than an hour each day can compromise immunity. This is a very powerful point to keep in mind.

It Will Jump-Start Your Brain

Aggravated about forgetting things? Want to jump-start your memory bank? Gerontology studies have conclusively demonstrated that as we age, we don't necessarily become more forgetful, scatterbrained, or ditsy. We sometimes do, however, process information at a slower rate. But this is certainly not the case for all older Americans. What keeps us and them sharp? You guessed it—the flip. Here is what the experts have to say:

- Dr. Kristine Yaffe, assistant professor of psychiatry and neurology at the University of California, San Francisco: "Exercise is good for cognitive function, which includes memory. Exercise also promotes attention and alertness, both of which are needed for encoding memories."

- Dr. Jay Lombard, assistant clinical professor of neurology at Cornell University's Medical College: "We need to reduce stress and increase antioxidant levels to counter the so-called natural aging of the brain."

- James Joseph, chief of neuroscience at Tufts University's Human Nutrition Research Center on Aging: "The brain needs its treasure trove of antioxidants—powerful chemicals that disarm free radicals, the harmful molecules created when the body converts food into energy and when it breaks down toxic substances."

A diet that is packed with fruits and vegetables will supply the necessary antioxidants. (As we discussed in Chapter 7, you are what you eat.) When free radicals are more prevalent in the body, they can contribute to a host of diseases and injure brain cells. In addition, as you age, your body's natural defenses weaken, which can allow free radicals to be more destructive. That's why, at any age, but even more so as we get older, a bountiful supply of antioxidants is vital.

Flipping: The Fountain of Youth for Your Brain

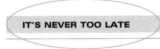

IT'S NEVER TOO LATE

Did you know that approximately 20 percent of your heart's output in blood goes straight to your brain? According to *Health* magazine, "a poorly functioning, failing heart does not supply the brain as it should and can result in a general clouding of thinking ability, memory and mental sharpness." Reducing body weight and performing strength and resistance exercise will help reduce stress, which has also been shown to impede memory. Therefore, the whole process of flipping can have a significant effect on your memory. Try this. Close the book right now. Do you remember most of the points I just made in this chapter? Do you remember what Billie Burke had to say about aging? Once you flip, you will.

You're not too old. It's never too late. Don't "act your age." Be any age you want to be.

PUTTING IT ALL TOGETHER TO FLIP

- Flipping is the equivalent of the fountain of youth when it comes to the aging process. Approximately one-third of the aging process is determined by your genes; the remainder is determined by your behavior.

- The functioning of the heart, the most important muscle in the body, can be significantly improved by coupling a low-calorie, plant-based (high in fruits and vegetables, with their powerful antioxidants) eating plan with intelligent strength and resistance exercise.

- Bone is active tissue. Strength and resistance exercise builds and maintains strong bones, thus minimizing the risk of osteoporosis.

- Lean muscle mass can be preserved and increased at any age by performing strength and resistance exercise.

- Individuals who flip can plan on living a far more independent lifestyle than those who don't.

- Exercise enhances mood through a variety of ways that can ease, if not completely eliminate, the effects of depression.

- Weight loss, coupled with strength and resistance exercise, minimizes many of the pains of aging such as arthritis.

- A diet high in antioxidants—one packed with fruits and vegetables—plus all of the positive mental and physical effects of strength and resistance exercise enhance memory and overall brain functioning.

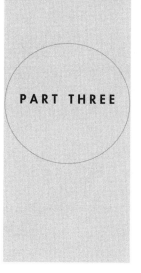

Living Flipped

11 "Oh No, I Just Gained Five Pounds Back," or How to Stay Flipped for Life

Diane Sawyer took a one-week vacation, then had an overwhelmingly difficult two weeks at work. She and I never worked out during that period, though we did stay in touch via e-mail and voice mail. The moment I saw her on the first day we worked out, she immediately blurted out, "Oh no, I gained five pounds back," to which I replied, "Good." She looked puzzled by my comment. I said, "Now you know what you can't do if you are going to stay flipped for life. Let's figure out what you did wrong—we know what you have been previously doing right—and let's get you right back on track."

She was relieved after we talked about it. In three weeks, Diane shed the five pounds. But this time, she lost that weight with more insight and understanding of what it means to stay flipped for life.

Here's a fact: Almost every person I know who has flipped has at some point gained some weight back. This happens for a variety of reasons:

- An extended vacation

- A "crunch" time in business

- A death in the family

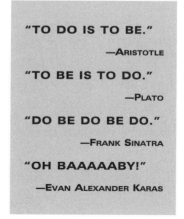

"TO DO IS TO BE."
—ARISTOTLE

"TO BE IS TO DO."
—PLATO

"DO BE DO BE DO."
—FRANK SINATRA

"OH BAAAAABY!"
—EVAN ALEXANDER KARAS

"OH NO, I JUST GAINED FIVE POUNDS BACK"

When I gain five pounds back, I feel . . .

_____

_____

_____

_____

_____

_____

_____

_____

_____

_____

_____

_____

_____

_____

_____

_____

_____

- An ill relative, friend, or spouse

- A celebration week

- A brief "lapse" in your belief that you can live flipped for life

Gaining Five Pounds Can Be *Good*

You know what I am talking about: *Everyone* has regained some weight after they flipped. Your first thought is, "Oh, forget it. All this hard work and I messed up. I'm just a failure." Sound familiar? Then the weight just continues to go up until you have gained back all the weight you lost and maybe even some more. But you must realize, gaining five pounds can be *good*. Yes, gaining some weight back gives you data regarding your behavior. After you gain some weight back, I want you to complete the following sentence: *When I gain five pounds back, I feel . . .* (Use the space provided at left.)

My response would be: *When I gain five pounds back, I feel so angry with myself. I knew my weight was going up, because I could see it in my face and around my waist. My jeans were uncomfortable, and I purposely avoided the scale because I was afraid of the reality. Then I got on. Oh yes, up five, maybe even more, pounds. Damn! If I'd just weighed myself sooner, I might have saved myself a few pounds.*

Does this sound like you? You knew you were overeating, or underexercising, or, most likely, both. Now you know that flipping is not a one-shot experience. Quite the contrary, it is something you will have to do over and over again for life.

Accept It: You Will Sometimes Fall Off the Wagon

SETBACKS ARE NATURAL AND MANAGEABLE

Carlo DiClemente, Ph.D., chairman of the psychology department at the University of Maryland in Baltimore, says, "The sooner you accept that falling off the wagon is likely, the greater your chances for long-term success. It's like learning to ride a bicycle. You just need to repeat the process until you (learn what you need to) get there." A relapse can actually make your next flip better planned, executed, and, most important, lasting. Why?

Behavior Has Consequences

First, you learn that what you have done has consequences. You have to go back and think, "Okay, if I gained five pounds, that means . . .":

I OVERATE BY HOW MANY CALORIES?
LET'S DO THE MATH: 3,500 CALORIES = 1 POUND, SO 3,500 CALORIES × 5 POUNDS = 17,500 CALORIES.

That's approximately how many calories you overate. When you think about it, you are probably lucky you regained only five pounds. It could easily have been more since you may have been really out of control. Just for the record, the reason you gained *only* five pounds was because you had previously increased your metabolism through strength and resistance exercise. Good thing you did that in the first place or just think of where you would be right now.

or

FLIPPING IS NOT A ONE-TIME DEAL

I STOPPED MAKING STRENGTH AND RESISTANCE EXERCISE A PRIORITY

Think back over the past few weeks. Was your strength and resistance exercise erratic? Did you miss many sessions? Were you working hard enough? Review your training log to obtain this data. Were you making exercise a priority? If you believe you can stay flipped for life and at some point cease strength and resistance exercise, then I have done an inadequate job of presenting my case. The only way to stay flipped for life is to perform strength and resistance training for life. Period.

Several years ago, I had a client in her early fifties who lost more than thirty pounds on my plan. She is the wife of an extremely overweight CEO in Chicago, so losing weight was a challenge given his eating habits. (I was at a cocktail party that included a children's sweets table, and I actually saw him eat two chocolate eclairs before hors d'oeuvres and dinner—yes, *before* hors d'oeuvres and dinner.) Together, they took a long weekend trip to Palm Springs to golf (his sport), play tennis (her sport), and relax with friends. When she returned, I arrived for our appointed exercise session and went up to meet her in her building's exercise room. She generally would be already there warming up. After waiting fifteen minutes (the doorman had called her, and she instructed him to send me to the exercise room, and she had never been late before for an appointment), I called her from my cell phone. I said, "Hey, is everything all right? I'm down here waiting and I am starting to get concerned." She said, "I just can't work out today. I am so depressed. I gained five pounds back. I'm so angry and disappointed with myself. I figured why even try. I'm going to take some time off from all this weight-loss stuff. Just charge me for today and send me a final bill."

I took a deep breath and said, "This is not unusual. To be perfectly honest, I expect all my clients to gain back some weight from time to time. I slip up from time to time myself and gain weight! We are all human. So stop feeling sorry for yourself and stop beating yourself up. You are only making matters worse. Put your shoes on, come down here, and let's get right back on track. You can't let one weekend sidetrack you from your goal." On the other end, after pause, pause, pause, I heard an inhale, then, "All right. I'm coming down."

Chips, Cheese, and Crackers

For the next hour, we did a little exercise and a lot of talking. She told me she'd had a great time on the trip and ate all the foods she loved, such as guacamole, chips, cheese, and crackers. Her host was a gourmet cook and "master of the Margarita" so it was margaritas every night. Eventually she did begin to laugh. She said it was just a domino effect: Everyone was eating and drinking and she just got caught up in it all. It sounded like fun to me. But when she returned home, the reality set in. Of course, you can have a great time, eat, drink, or whatever, but don't go crazy. Remember, you are in the weight-loss game for life. And for the record, vacation does not have to mean that you totally forget your flip.

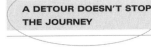

A DETOUR DOESN'T STOP THE JOURNEY

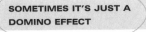

SOMETIMES IT'S JUST A DOMINO EFFECT

Spin Yourself Back to the Flip

I know what you're saying. Each of you is shaking your head and thinking, "Well, she had Jim Karas to get her back on track. I don't have anyone to help me. That's why I fail." No, no, no. You do have someone to help you get back on track—you. Yes, *you*. You have the power to spin yourself back to the flip. You did it once, you can do it again.

YOU HAVE THE POWER

Take the Flip on the Road

Here's an idea. Let's say you're getting ready to go away for a long weekend—maybe it's a family reunion, a trip for some sun, or a time to take the kids to Disney World. You know it's going to be rough. First, make sure to pack your exercise clothes and any portable exercise equipment, such as the SPRI Xertubes or Xerings.

Forget the dumbbells; select easy-to-pack exercise equipment. As you plan your trip, call ahead to see if where you will be staying has an exercise facility; today most hotels do, and some even have personal trainers on staff. If an exercise facility is not on the premises, see if the management can recommend one that is nearby. If there is no facility in the area, don't worry. You can use a jump rope and your SPRI Xertubes and Xerings in your room. Even if you get in only ten or fifteen minutes a day, that's better than no exercise at all. The important thing is to make exercise a priority, even though you are on vacation. Schedule it; plan for it. Say to your friends, spouse, kids, whoever is joining you or meeting you on the trip that each day you are going to take some time for *yourself* and exercise. Once again, it's your vacation as well as theirs. Why not take some of that time and put it to good use? Use the time for you.

Unfortunately, the opposite often occurs. Frequently, because you are on a trip, your schedule is more hectic than ever. Everyone wants to do something different. You are worried about everyone having a good time, being able to do what they want to do, and end up totally overlooking your own needs. I stressed this a great deal in Chapter 3, "'I Don't Have the Time,'" but it warrants repeating: If you take the time to exercise, regardless of whether you are at home or on vacation, it will make you happier, calmer, less stressed, and less depressed,

MAKE TIME FOR YOURSELF WHEN YOU'RE ON THE ROAD

and provide you with a sense of accomplishment. This is bad? Of course not. If you take some time to exercise and to take care of yourself, then everyone, including you, benefits.

There's No Vacation from the Flip

A lot of you will decide that vacation is the time to take off from exercise. I have had dozens, if not hundreds, of conversations like this one with my clients:

Me: "So, you're going away for a week. Are you taking your exercise clothes and shoes?"

Client: "No way! This is my vacation. I'm taking the week off."

Me: "Okay, just realize going in that the odds are if you don't exercise for one week and do your 'vacation' eating, you are without a doubt going to gain weight. Exercise during the trip and you will minimize the damage. The choice is yours. What will it be?"

The client gives me a blank stare and mutters something.

So, exercise when you are out of town, whether you are away for business or pleasure. Please. You know how strongly I believe in strength and resistance exercise, but use the time away to take some great walks along a beach, explore a new city on foot, or hike in the mountains. Run around with the kids, snow or water ski, rent a bike, do anything that helps burn a few additional calories while you're away. It will make all the difference when you return to reality.

Traveler's Advisory: Avoid Taking an Eating Vacation

Eating on vacation does not give you license to go wild. Pace yourself. Apply many of the eating rules I gave you in Chapter 7. Sample the local foods, but first ask how they are prepared. And don't forget, portion control still applies. If you are vacationing in a warm climate, odds are that fruits and vegetables will be plentiful and fresh, so enjoy. Again, it's all part of deciding what you want for yourself and your life.

What Undid Your Flip?

A trip can be easily managed. You can plan for it. In the scheme of things, a trip is easy to work around. Unfortunately, other factors are

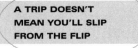

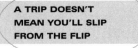

A TRIP DOESN'T MEAN YOU'LL SLIP FROM THE FLIP

less easy to identify and manage. Reflect on what's taking place in your life. What has changed? Are you under stress? Depressed? Maybe you didn't get asked out by that guy you like at the coffee shop. I don't know. Only you can answer these questions. In most cases, you will be able to pinpoint the event or situation that undid your flip. You need to determine whether it was a physical factor that unflipped you, such as a business or pleasure trip, or an emotional factor, such as the loss of a loved one.

For many years, I didn't ask this question in an initial consultation with a new client. Subsequently, I realized that this was one of the most important questions, because something happened almost every time that caused the weight gain. You need to identify this factor and deal with it. If you gained the weight because you moved and never got around to joining a heath club or gym nearby, then scout the gyms nearby and make the decision to join one. If you gained weight because you are nursing an ill spouse or parent, then realize that this is a time when you need more energy and strength than ever before. Flip again, and you will be better able to cope with any difficult situation.

STAY IN TOUCH WITH YOUR EMOTIONAL AND PHYSICAL CHANGES

Ask Yourself, "How Am I Feeling About My Body?"

One tool that I have successfully employed with clients over the years to keep them on track is to ask them every month or so how they are feeling about their bodies. If you recall, I urged you to ask yourself

"OH NO, I JUST GAINED FIVE POUNDS BACK"

My current impression of my body is . . .

_____

_____

_____

_____

_____

_____

_____

_____

_____

_____

_____

_____

_____

_____

_____

_____

_____

the same question in Chapter 1. Constant monitoring of your current attitude toward your body is essential. As you continue the process of flipping, you need to stay in touch with the emotional and physical changes that are also taking place: kids, divorce, getting older, health, elderly parents, career, and so on. This can be accomplished if on the first of every month you complete the following sentence: _My current impression of my body is . . ._ (Use the space provided at left.)

As I've already recommended, you need to complete this sentence on a monthly basis. (See the worksheets in the back of this book.) As you are recording your progress each month, you can gauge whether things are getting out of hand. If you notice a negative tone creeping into your positive entries, or that you have been omitting entries and not performing this exercise monthly, then you should be alert to make the necessary corrections to keep yourself from losing your flip and allowing old feelings, impressions, and behaviors to prevail.

It Happens to Everyone

As I wrote this chapter, I discussed the issue of gaining five pounds back with others. You need to realize that this happens to everyone. I recently attended yet another birthday party with my daughter. At the party, I spoke with a few of the very thin moms, the kind of women you would think would _never_ put on extra pounds. They became totally animated about the subject of gaining weight back. These thirty- and forty-something mothers regaled me with stories about chocolate attacks that lasted for five days; eating all the Easter candy _before_ the big holiday and having to buy more for the kids; love affairs with carmel corn; "Big Mac" attacks—you name it. They were really funny as each one tried to trump the other with her eating story.

My wife, Ellen, who has never had a weight problem, said to me a couple of weeks after Halloween, "You have to remove all Snickers from the house. I'm out of control. I just can't stop eating them." (For the record, we gave out Snickers for Halloween and these were the leftovers. I bet you thought I'd be handing out carrot sticks.) *Everyone* who overeats or underexercises experiences that five-pound weight gain multiple times in his or her life. This applies to *all* individuals— fat, thin, tall, short, young, old, male, female—including the wives of weight-loss professionals.

The key to coping with these setbacks is awareness. You need to be aware of this behavior before it gets too far out of hand and negates all the good work you have done. This is what separates the losers from the *losers*. You cannot allow a minor setback to pull you permanently off course. Believe me, it really is only a minor setback, not the beginning of the end unless you allow it to be. You have in your possession the tools to regain your focus and, once again, believe in your ability to continue the flip. Here are a few additional suggestions to facilitate your flip.

> **EVEN THIN PEOPLE CAN GAIN WEIGHT—IT HAPPENS IN MY HOUSE**

Trust the Scale

You have to weigh yourself once every week. I know that some people tell you, "Stop being a slave to the scale. What's important is how you feel, not what a scale has to say." That could not be further from the truth. The scale is the data. The scale tells you, whether you like it or not, what is going on with your body. Recently, a prospective client called my office. One of the questions each of my staff is instructed to ask is the current height and weight of the individual. Let's face it, we are in the business of helping people lose weight, so it's not in any way inappropriate for us to ask. The woman on the other line said something like "How dare you. I would never discuss my weight with someone I don't know." My staff member had enough sense to place the woman on hold and ask me, "What do I do?" I said, "I'll take it." I picked up the phone and said, "Hi, this is Jim Karas. We are so excited that you are interested in working with my firm. I want to personally finish your client-intake information form with you. Now, what is your present height and weight?" There was silence.

Finally, she said, "I really have to apologize for what I said to the gentleman on the phone. The truth is, I haven't weighed myself in years. It's too scary. I know I have gained a lot of weight. I was just too embarrassed to tell him that."

I believe her. I believe most individuals I have come across who state that they haven't been on the scale in years, and that even includes the doctor's office when they get their physical exams. If you are going to a doctor who lets you decide whether you are weighed or not, it's time to get a new doctor. The purpose of a physical exam is to provide data. Your body weight is one of those important pieces of data. Body weight is a necessary piece of information in order to prescribe the appropriate amount of a medication.

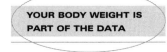
YOUR BODY WEIGHT IS PART OF THE DATA

Same Day, Same Time, Same Scale

The rules that apply to the scale are simple: You weigh yourself on the same scale at the same time on the same day each week. Please don't pop on your neighbor's scale, or a hotel room scale, or the one at the club if that is not the one you are regularly using. The best scales are the balance-beam scales similar to the ones you are weighed on at a doctor's office. You may notice that you always weigh more on that scale. Why? Well, that scale is correct and the one you are using at home is most likely incorrect. But the one at home is the control (in other words, it's always the same), so stick with the numbers you see on that scale. Keep in mind that most likely your scale is anywhere from three to seven pounds "light." That's right. Unless you own a doctor's office–quality balance-beam scale, you probably weigh three to seven pounds more than what your home scale is telling you. Don't get mad at me. Don't be frightened by this fact. On the contrary, feel informed.

Blast or Bust?

I have one more story to tell about my wife, since you need to realize that even the people who live with me sometimes gain weight. Ellen played Mary Haines in the Arena Stage production of *The Women* in Washington, D.C. Our good friend Kyle Donnelly (she is the reason Ellen and I met) was the director. Before they left for three months, she said to Ellen, "Well, with eighteen women working together, this is going to be either a blast or a bust." Well, it was a blast. The gals really enjoyed the play and carried the party long into the evenings. After the first few performances, they celebrated with champagne. Then they added food. Then they started baking. Boy, were they having a good time! As I would see the show once every other week, I experienced firsthand the cast's "expansion."

So, a "bloated" version of Ellen came home after three months. On the first morning back, she started to put on a pair of pants, threw them down, and told me, "The dry cleaner shrunk my pants." Then she tried on a pair of jeans and said, "Someone must have put these into the dryer." I said nothing, which as you may know by now, is rare. Finally, after the fifth day of her throwing clothes down and blaming everyone else, I said *very* diplomatically, "You might want to pop on the scale." She sent me an icy glare and walked into the bathroom. After a great deal of banging on the balance-beam scale, she came out and said, "I can't believe it. This couldn't have happened. I've gained over ten pounds. I'm horrified!" Had she jumped on the scale sooner, she would have known sooner. For the record, she was back down to flipped weight in about four weeks.

Try on Your Clothes

In Chapter 2, "Visualize the Flip," I instructed you to try on old clothing every month. In the beginning, I wanted you to perform this exercise to motivate you to once again be able to fit into some of the clothing that you once wore at a lower body weight. Now I want you to do it to make sure you *stay* at your current successfully flipped body weight. Clothes don't lie (Ellen's didn't) just as a scale doesn't lie. You and I know that. Keep trying them on, keep looking and feeling great, always increase your awareness of what's happening, and you won't lose your flip.

Face the Fear and It Will Disappear

You did it before and you can do it again. Once a month, take a good, hard look at your body in a full-length mirror. See before your eyes all the great changes your body has made. I often hear women talk

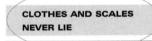

CLOTHES AND SCALES
NEVER LIE

about the new definition they see in their arms, their reshaped rear ends, and the disappearance of cellulite. The men talk about flat abs, decent pecs, and strong legs.

If you promise yourself that on the first of every month you will do a little "mirror" inventory, you will be able to see if you are moving forward or falling back. Trust the mirror, the scale, and the clothing. These are some of your best tools when it comes to staying successfully flipped. It's also motivating to look great—it's positive aesthetic reinforcement.

To review, I want you to:

- Once a month, complete the sentence "My current impression of my body is . . ."

- Once a week, weigh yourself on the same scale, on the same day, at the same time.

- Once a month, try on your flipped clothes and feel how they fit.

- Once a month, take a few minutes to look at your body in a full-length mirror. Evaluate the changes, good or bad.

None of this is being narcissistic. This is being focused. Believe me, it works.

Children, Menopause, and the Flip Revisited

For women, it is necessary to once again address childbirth and menopause, because they can have such a significant impact on a woman's behavior and weight. Both of these factors cause the Balance of Energy Equation to shift. For one, carrying a baby requires you to gain weight—there is no way around it. But you cannot allow this wonderful experience to

CAN CELLULITE DISAPPEAR?

Based on my experience, the appearance of cellulite can be minimized with weight loss. I use the word *minimize* because, for some, cellulite cannot be completely eliminated. Strength and resistance exercise is the best form of exercise to reduce the appearance of cellulite. While I do not believe in "spot toning," strengthening the muscles in an area can slightly hold the body fat in more tightly, and if you reduce the amount of fat on your body, you'll consequently reduce the amount of cellulite. Many female clients have told me that they see the difference with my program and the results of the strength and resistance exercise.

be clouded by the fact that you have to gain weight. Many women express their fear to me. They say, "What am I going to do? I worked so hard to lose the weight in the first place. Now I have to gain it all back." To which I reply, "This is only a temporary situation. Your responsibility right now is to carry a healthy baby, maintain your lean muscle tissue, keep exercising, eat healthy foods to fuel your body and the baby's body, and minimize the weight gain. My responsibility is to make sure that happens.

"Remember, this time you are gaining the weight for the baby, not for your hips and thighs. Does that sound so hard?" My clients' reply is almost always the same: "No, but I'm still nervous." Most of these women gain between twenty and thirty pounds with the baby and leave the hospital with between twelve and fifteen pounds of excess weight. In no time, that weight is lost and they are at their prepregnancy weight, with lean muscle tissue preserved, metabolism maintained, energy level up (which every new mom knows is beneficial with a newborn), and the belief that once again they can stay flipped for life. Why was the weight loss relatively easy? They had boosted their metabolism through strength and resistance exercise and knew how to count their calories. They basically stayed flipped throughout their pregnancy. It sounds like a tall order, but it's much easier than you think. Believe it, you can stay flipped and have children—living flipped and having children are not incompatible.

Going through menopause and staying flipped is more difficult. You may find that what you were doing to lose or maintain weight loss is not enough once you enter menopause. I said this before, but I feel it requires repeating: Once you enter menopause, your old weight-*loss* behavior may become your new weight-*maintenance* behavior. To lose weight, you have to fine-tune even further.

Diet or Super-Diet?

Many clients have told me that once they entered menopause, they had to always "diet" to maintain their weight and "super-diet" to lose any weight. From my experience, they are correct. Sorry, I don't want to depress you, but I do want you to be knowledgeable. Middle age does not mean being overweight. Your age has nothing to do with your weight. Behavior determines your weight.

What about men, pregnancy, and menopause? It is essential that you, too, understand what is going on so that you can be compassionate with your partner when she goes through these changes. Once the baby is born, encourage your wife or partner to exercise (offer to baby-sit to give her some time), eat low-calorie foods (make sure they're on hand—she may not have the opportunity to shop for them), and convince her that you still find her sexy and attractive. Flip with her and both of you will look and feel better. When your spouse, friend, or family member enters menopause, show her that you understand at least a part of what she is going through. Cite some of the information I have discussed throughout this book. Be empathetic. This is not fun for her. You may be able to make it a little better if you can be supportive. And if you decide to flip with her, you then both look better, feel better, possess more energy, and, most likely, increase your life span together. That sounds like a win-win situation to me.

This is the time when you really have to establish a plan. Don't despair. Just realize that the rules change somewhat after menopause, and I want you to be ready and prepared for that change. I have helped hundreds, if not thousands, of women during this time and many of them have lost weight and inches, and feel in the best shape of their lives. So can you. Go back and look at Chapter 9 for more information and support on staying flipped during menopause.

Men and the Flip

Just because men don't go through menopause and don't bear children, that doesn't mean that they, too, don't gain weight. Most gain a considerable amount of weight starting in their forties and fifties. Why? Without regular strength and resistance exercise, men lose those calorie-burning muscles just as women do. This leads to a reduced metabolism and subsequent weight gain. Men tend to overeat, drink alcohol more than women, and watch more television than women. This all causes the Balance of Energy Equation to favor weight gain. Men have just as much to gain from the flip as women do.

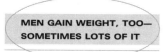

MEN GAIN WEIGHT, TOO—
SOMETIMES LOTS OF IT

Victory

I have a good friend who was really feeling low one day. He had been successful in many areas of his life, but that was in the past. As we were talking one day, he said, "You know, right now, I just need another victory." I found that comment interesting. It made me think. All of us have had some sort of victory in our past. It might have been getting a job we really wanted, going on a date with someone we liked for a long time, finding the perfect gift for a friend, or having scored the winning goal.

Couldn't you use a victory right now? We all can at any point in our lives. Maybe you are staying at home with young kids and thinking, "How am I going to get through the next ten years?" or sitting at your office after having been passed over for the promotion you know you deserved and wondering, "How am I going to keep myself from getting really, really depressed and angry about this situation?" or leaving a clothing store once again unable to find anything that fits and figuring, "I might as well stop at the House of Pies and pick up dinner."

This doesn't have to be you. You can flip right now—that's right, *right now.* You can take control of your health and appearance. Doing so will produce a glorious victory. You can throw this book down, stand up, and proclaim, "I'm going to do it. I'm going to flip the switch." Shut your office door or find a moment of privacy in your home, then look into a mirror and say, "I'm going to do it." I know it's tough, but the tougher and more truthful you are, the better your chances are of staying flipped for life. Life is filled with choices— make one of those choices to be victorious with your weight loss.

Get Tough

According to the *Tufts University Heath & Nutrition Letter,* "the stricter the diet and the more weight loss, the more weight that's kept off." I have always found this to be true. If you asked me, "What is the common denominator that most individuals possess when it comes to a successful flip?" I would respond, "Consistency, documentation, and an ongoing belief in one's ability to stay flipped for

YOU CAN START TO
FLIP RIGHT NOW

life." In other words, a well-thought-out approach and a clear adherence to the plan. Why? The answer to that is simple. If you approach your plan in an unfocused way, you are going to achieve *unfocused* results, which are not very motivating. But if you approach your plan with a clear belief that you will succeed, follow through, and adhere to the plan, then you will achieve great results, which are motivating. If the scale moves down just a little bit, you think, "All this work and I lose only a half pound in three weeks." That's not very motivating. But if you *really* do it, *really* get serious with your food and your exercise plan, the scale will *really* move. The clothes get looser. Comments such as "What are you doing? You look just great!" keep coming at you. These are the motivators that keep you flipped for life, because they reinforce your internal belief in your ability to successfully flip.

"I Did It Before, I Can Do It Again"

I always try to impress upon people that if they've been successful at weight loss in the past, they will be in the future. Please know that I am not saying that you have to eat celery and carrots for the rest of your life and never touch another cookie. That could not be further from the truth. But you must understand that you have the control in this matter. You control what goes into your mouth. No one can force you to eat. You decide what you want to eat. No one can prohibit you from exercising. You decide whether or not to exercise. If you gain five pounds back, make a clear decision that you are going to get that weight off once again. Believe in yourself. You can do it! Tell yourself, "I did it before, I can do it again. I did it before, I can do it again."

Look at it this way. You are up against some formidable opposition as you attempt to stay flipped. Your body continues to age. Without regular strength and resistance exercise you continue to lose lean muscle tissue, which can slow your metabolism. As you age, the tendency is to become more sedentary, which will reduce the calories out in your Balance of Energy Equation. We know that food is more readily available—it's everywhere, all around us. We watch TV more, sit at a computer more, walk less, drive more. As you get older, you may be more financially successful, which affords you the opportunity to

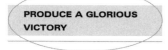

PRODUCE A GLORIOUS VICTORY

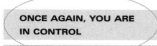

ONCE AGAIN, YOU ARE IN CONTROL

eat in restaurants more often, buy prepared foods, and travel more than in the past. All of these factors and more may play havoc with and thwart your ability to stay flipped. Notice that I said "may." Only you can decide if you will allow it. You have to want to flip. If you don't want to do it, trust me, it won't happen.

The Response Factor

The response you receive from people regarding your success is yet another issue. You will be amazed. It's quite interesting how individuals respond to the success of others, even close friends.

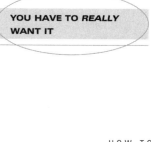

YOU HAVE TO *REALLY* WANT IT

Undoubtedly you will find people close to you who say nothing about the obvious physical, and most likely psychological, changes that have occurred as a result of your successful flip. A friend can be sitting next to you at a dinner, when an acquaintance comes up and exclaims, "You look great. What have you been doing?" After a few minutes more of praise and a discussion of your obvious change, the individual who has been complimenting your success leaves. The friend sitting next to you doesn't say a word. As you think about it, this person has never remarked on your successful flip. You start to wonder if you are doing something wrong.

On the contrary, you are doing something so very right that it is difficult for some people to acknowledge and accept it. If you succeed at weight loss when statistically we know that so many fail, then your achievement singles you out. That is threatening to some people. Most likely, it will highlight the fact that others are doing something wrong. Also, many individuals who are unhappy with themselves are envious of others. They refuse to shoulder the blame for their poor food and exercise behavior. "Oh no," you're thinking, "that would never happen to me. My friends and colleagues wouldn't respond like that." Trust me, they will. Be prepared for people to try to unflip you with remarks such as, "You're just getting obsessive with this diet and exercise," "I bet all you do is work out and eat carrots all day," "If I had the time, I could do it, but I am just too busy," and "Act your age and stop trying to stay so young."

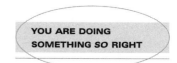

YOU ARE DOING SOMETHING *SO* RIGHT

I Struggle, You Struggle, We All Struggle

Losing weight is tough. I work on it every day. I struggle with my weight just as much as the next person. At any moment, if I ease up, I know I will gain some weight back. Most people assume I have always been at my present weight. I wish this were the case, but, as you know by now, unfortunately it isn't. Yes, yes, yes, I struggle with my weight *all the time.* That shocks people. Most individuals who have never lost weight think that you only have to flip once—that once you lose weight, you're done. You and I know that is very far from the truth. Flipping is a lifelong process. Try to put your friends' or colleagues' hurtful remarks in context. Perhaps even offer to help them by explaining the ideas behind *Flip the Switch* and giving them their own copy. Once you lose weight, you become a role model for successful weight loss. Realize that you are stepping into that position. You're informed. Share your knowledge with others when asked. You don't want to irritate people, just be polite *when asked.*

Think back to the first chapter of this book where I urged you to believe in your ability to succeed at weight loss. Don't be afraid to believe in the power of yourself. Believing in yourself will create a life-changing opportunity. By doing so, you will be creating a foundation upon which to build success in all areas of your life, not only weight loss.

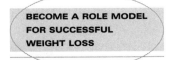

BECOME A ROLE MODEL FOR SUCCESSFUL WEIGHT LOSS

Remember Anne?

Go back to the first page of the introduction to this book, where dietitian Anne Fletcher stated that for individuals who had successfully flipped, the desire to lose weight finally became more important than the desire to overeat and not to exercise. Ask yourself, "Has my desire to lose weight become more important than my desire to overeat and not to exercise?" If the answer to that question is no, then you need to return to the introduction and read this book again. I hope reading it helped you to understand many of the complex physical and psychological components of flipping. I also hope that reading *Flip the Switch* has given you the information you need to successfully lose weight, even if you choose not to do so at this point in your life. It's possible that this book has awakened many strong emotions or feelings that you have kept bottled up inside. Now you know you have to overcome these painful issues and prevent them from being a barrier to your success. I know that you won't be able to successfully flip for life until you explore all the factors that have led you to gain the weight. Only then can you undertake the process of losing the weight.

The "Fat Suit"

For many, added weight is like an armor or shield. For some, it's their "fat suit." As long as you have the armor or fat suit on, no one can hurt you and get to what is beneath the shield. As long as the fat suit is on, no one can see *you*. It becomes such as part of you that the thought of taking it off is scary. That is where the "desire" that Anne Fletcher refers to must stem from. You have to be ready to take the fat suit off and reveal the real *you*. The problem is, if you haven't done any work on *you*, then the likelihood that you will allow others to see the real *you* is small.

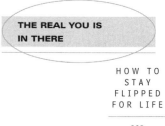

THE REAL YOU IS
IN THERE

HOW TO
STAY
FLIPPED
FOR LIFE

293

Flip from the Inside Out

Once again, most people attempt weight loss from the outside in. I urge you to attempt weight loss *from the inside out.* That is why I started this book with "Believe in the Flip." First, prepare emotionally for the challenge and believe you can do it, then muster the strength to meet the challenge, plan your strategy for attack, and meet the flip head-on.

In Chapter 1, I discussed the fact that change is scary. You may not be happy at your present weight, but the thought of losing weight (change) is harder than living with your present weight. That's somewhat shocking, but in so many instances it's true. If you consciously choose not to lose weight, fine. I don't want you to feel that I am imposing my beliefs on you. But if you are not happy with your present situation (which reading this book would tend to indicate), then emotionally prepare for the changes that are going to take place. You need to determine if this is the right time to remove your armor or that fat suit and embark on what for many will be a life-changing journey. The probability is high that you've previously attempted to lose weight. Unfortunately, the likelihood that you were unsuccessful is also high. I know that you are afraid of failing again. But now the situation is different. You've just read *Flip the Switch* and you possess the knowledge to turn your desire to lose weight into a reality. I have given you the road map. Only you can decide if you choose to follow it. I can guarantee that the change produced is a positive one: Once you've flipped, you will look better and feel better. All the uncertainty surrounding this change has been eliminated.

Listen to the Boys

We're coming toward the end of our journey. I opened this chapter with one of my favorite series of quotes. I wanted to use them in my first book, *The Business Plan for the Body*, but they didn't seem to fit. However, this time they do.

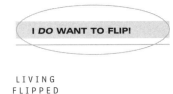

Remember what they were? "To do is to be": I think by this Aristotle meant, *Hey, you do it, you become it.* In other words, if you decide to flip the switch, you will become *it.* Recall Diane Sawyer getting her "it" back. You *will* become a weight loss success. Plato said, "To be is to do." *To be,* as in to be a weight-loss success, you have to *do it.* If you don't try to lose weight, it won't happen. There is no way to *be* if you don't *do.* And Frank Sinatra comes along with "Do be do be do." No doubt, the "Chairman of the Board" never expected his famous phrasing to wind up on these pages, but I don't just hear crooning, I hear "do" versus "be." This is the "mental graffiti" I've mentioned throughout this book. In your mind, you are on the fence. You are thinking about flipping and saying to yourself, "Do I? Don't I? Do I? Don't I?" My goal is for you to stop at the "Do I?" reverse it to "I Do," eliminate the question mark, and place a resounding exclamation point at the end. Say to yourself, "I Do Want to Flip!" and stop there.

That is what this book is all about. It's about getting to that point of feeling positive about yourself and your ability to succeed. Look back at each of the exercises I asked you to complete. Reread the sentences you've completed. Review your food and exercise journals.

Know that only you can make this decision. We flip a switch almost every time we enter a room at night. We flip a switch when we set an alarm clock. We flip a switch every time we turn on a television set. Now, rather than for light, a "wake-up call," or entertainment, this time *flip a switch for yourself.* Do it for your health, your mind, your family, your friends. But most of all, do it just for you.

I've loved taking you on this journey. I feel so positive that you have experienced mental growth and now have the sound knowledge to succeed at weight loss. My eighteen-month-old son, Evan, loves to squeal, "Oh baaaaaby!" whenever he sees himself in a mirror. You will say exactly the same thing after you flip the switch and lose the weight. I know you can do it. I've helped so many people to succeed at weight loss—Diane, Gayle, Dawnnie, and myself included—so come join us. Turn your weight loss desire into a reality. Close your eyes and repeat with me,

"IF THEY CAN DO IT, SO CAN I."

"IF THEY CAN DO IT, SO CAN I."

"IF THEY CAN DO IT, SO CAN I."

"IF THEY CAN DO IT, SO CAN I."

"IF THEY CAN DO IT, SO CAN I."

"IF THEY CAN DO IT, SO CAN I."

"IF THEY CAN DO IT, SO CAN I."

"IF THEY CAN DO IT, SO CAN I."

Monthly Inventory
Worksheets

JANUARY: Today's Date_____

Weight (record weekly)

DATE	AMOUNT
_____	_____
_____	_____
_____	_____
_____	_____

This Month, my current impression of my body is:

_____

_____

_____

_____

_____

This month, my clothes fit this way:

_____

_____

_____

_____

_____

This month, I feel this way about my progress so far:

_____

_____

_____

_____

_____

FEBRUARY: Today's Date_____

Weight (record weekly)

DATE	AMOUNT
————	————
————	————
————	————
————	————

This Month, my current impression of my body is:

_____

_____

_____

_____

_____

_____

This month, my clothes fit this way:

_____

_____

_____

_____

_____

This month, I feel this way about my progress so far:

_____

_____

_____

_____

_____

MARCH: Today's Date_____

Weight (record weekly)

DATE	AMOUNT
....	....
....	....
....	....
....	....

This Month, my current impression of my body is:

_____

_____

_____

_____

_____

This month, my clothes fit this way:

_____

_____

_____

_____

_____

This month, I feel this way about my progress so far:

_____

_____

_____

_____

_____

_____

APRIL: Today's Date_____

Weight (record weekly)

<table>
<tr><td></td><td>DATE</td><td>AMOUNT</td></tr>
<tr><td></td><td>_____</td><td>_____</td></tr>
<tr><td></td><td>_____</td><td>_____</td></tr>
<tr><td></td><td>_____</td><td>_____</td></tr>
<tr><td></td><td>_____</td><td>_____</td></tr>
</table>

This Month, my current impression of my body is:

_____

_____

_____

_____

_____

This month, my clothes fit this way:

_____

_____

_____

_____

_____

This month, I feel this way about my progress so far:

_____

_____

_____

_____

_____

MAY: Today's Date_____

Weight (record weekly)

DATE	AMOUNT
....	....
....	....
....	....
....	....

This Month, my current impression of my body is:

_____

_____

_____

_____

_____

This month, my clothes fit this way:

_____

_____

_____

_____

_____

This month, I feel this way about my progress so far:

_____

_____

_____

_____

_____

_____

JUNE: Today's Date_____

Weight (record weekly)

This Month, my current impression of my body is:

_____

_____

_____

_____

_____

This month, my clothes fit this way:

_____

_____

_____

_____

_____

This month, I feel this way about my progress so far:

_____

_____

_____

_____

_____

JULY: Today's Date_____

Weight (record weekly)

DATE	AMOUNT
————	————
————	————
————	————
————	————

This Month, my current impression of my body is:

_____

_____

_____

_____

_____

_____

This month, my clothes fit this way:

_____

_____

_____

_____

_____

_____

This month, I feel this way about my progress so far:

_____

_____

_____

_____

_____

_____

AUGUST: Today's Date_____

Weight (record weekly)

DATE	AMOUNT

This Month, my current impression of my body is:

_____

_____

_____

_____

_____

_____

This month, my clothes fit this way:

_____

_____

_____

_____

_____

This month, I feel this way about my progress so far:

_____

_____

_____

_____

_____

_____

SEPTEMBER: Today's Date_____

Weight (record weekly)

DATE	AMOUNT
_____	_____
_____	_____
_____	_____
_____	_____

This Month, my current impression of my body is:

_____

_____

_____

_____

_____

_____

This month, my clothes fit this way:

_____

_____

_____

_____

_____

_____

This month, I feel this way about my progress so far:

_____

_____

_____

_____

_____

_____

OCTOBER: Today's Date_____

Weight (record weekly)

DATE	AMOUNT
————	————
————	————
————	————
————	————

This Month, my current impression of my body is:

_____

_____

_____

_____

_____

This month, my clothes fit this way:

_____

_____

_____

_____

_____

This month, I feel this way about my progress so far:

_____

_____

_____

_____

_____

NOVEMBER: Today's Date_____

Weight (record weekly)

DATE	AMOUNT
_____	_____
_____	_____
_____	_____
_____	_____

This Month, my current impression of my body is:

_____

_____

_____

_____

_____

_____

This month, my clothes fit this way:

_____

_____

_____

_____

_____

_____

This month, I feel this way about my progress so far:

_____

_____

_____

_____

_____

_____

DECEMBER: Today's Date_____

Weight (record weekly)

DATE	AMOUNT
....	....
....	....
....	....
....	....

This Month, my current impression of my body is: _____

_____

_____

_____

_____

_____

This month, my clothes fit this way: _____

_____

_____

_____

_____

_____

This month, I feel this way about my progress so far: _____

_____

_____

_____

_____

_____

_____

DAILY FOOD DIARY

Date_____

Meal	Food/Beverage Consumed	Amount	Calories	Comments
Breakfast				
Snack				
Lunch				
Snack				
Dinner				
Snack				
Water				
	Total			
	Over/Under Against Daily Calories			

PROGRAM ONE: SPRI TUBING AND RESIST-A-BALL

Date_____

Exercise		Mon	Tues	Wed	Thurs	Fri	Sat	Sun
Seated Back Rows on Ball	Lbs/Tubes							
	Reps							
Rear Deltoid Fly on Ball	Lbs/Tubes							
	Reps							
Seated Chest Press on Ball	Lbs/Tubes							
	Reps							
Standing Bicep Curl	Lbs/Tubes							
	Reps							
Tricep Pushdown	Lbs/Tubes							
	Reps							
Hip Extension	Lbs/Tubes							
	Reps							
Hip Abduction	Lbs/Tubes							
	Reps							
Side Steps with Xering	Lbs/Tubes							
	Reps							
Ball Wall Squats	Lbs/Tubes							
	Reps							
Abs with Xertube	Lbs/Tubes							
	Reps							

FLIP THE SWITCH STRENGTH AND RESISTANCE TRAINING LOG

PROGRAM TWO: FREE WEIGHTS AND RESIST-A-BALL

Date_____

Exercise		Mon	Tues	Wed	Thurs	Fri	Sat	Sun
One Arm Row	Lbs/Tubes							
	Reps							
Chest Press with Ball	Lbs/Tubes							
	Reps							
Bicep Curl	Lbs/Tubes							
	Reps							
Tricep Extension	Lbs/Tubes							
	Reps							
Rear Deltoid Fly	Lbs/Tubes							
	Reps							
Dead Lift	Lbs/Tubes							
	Reps							
Squat	Lbs/Tubes							
	Reps							
Stationary Lunge	Lbs/Tubes							
	Reps							
Hamstring Curl on Ball	Lbs/Tubes							
	Reps							
Abs on the Ball	Lbs/Tubes							
	Reps							

FLIP THE SWITCH **STRENGTH AND RESISTANCE TRAINING LOG**

PROGRAM THREE: GYM WORKOUT

Date_____

Exercise		Mon	Tues	Wed	Thurs	Fri	Sat	Sun
Lat Pulldown	Lbs/Tubes							
	Reps							
Back Row	Lbs/Tubes							
	Reps							
Chest Press	Lbs/Tubes							
	Reps							
Bicep Curl	Lbs/Tubes							
	Reps							
Tricep Pushdown	Lbs/Tubes							
	Reps							
Leg Press	Lbs/Tubes							
	Reps							
Hamstring Curl	Lbs/Tubes							
	Reps							
Hip Extension	Lbs/Tubes							
	Reps							
Hip Abduction	Lbs/Tubes							
	Reps							
The Plank	Lbs/Tubes							
	Reps							

Resource Notes

CHAPTER 1

Chicago Tribune, November 18, 2001

New York Post, January 22, 2002

Nutrition Action Newsletter, March 2002, page 8

Parenting

Shape, October 1999, page 22; March 2002, page 118

Sills, Judith, Ph.D., *Excess Baggage,* Viking, 1993

USA Today, January 10, 2002, page 8D

Wall Street Journal, May 1, 2000, page R4

CHAPTER 2

Covey, Stephen, *The Seven Habits of Highly Effective People,* Simon & Schuster, 1990

Dahlkoetter, JoAnn, Ph.D., *Your Performing Edge,* Pulgas Ridge, 2002

Fitness, February 2002, page 70

CHAPTER 3

Consumer Reports on Health, November 2000

IDEA Health & Fitness Source, February 2000, page 31

CHAPTER 4

Ace Fitness Matters, Nov/Dec 2001, page 5

Chicago Magazine, February 2002, page 66

Chicago Tribune, September 23, 2001, section 13, page 2

Consumer Reports on Health, November 2000

Environmental Nutrition, September 2001

IDEA Health & Fitness Source, September 2001, pages 27–29

IDEA Personal Trainer, February 2002

Journal of the American Medical Association, September 12, 2001

The Lerner Publication—Skyline, June 15, 2000

Mayo Clinic Health Letter, October 2001

Newsweek, Special Issue, Fall/Winter 2001, page 33

Nutrition Action Healthletter, December 2001, page 9

Shape, March 2002, page 135

CHAPTER 5

Worth, May 2002, page 24

CHAPTER 6

Chicago Tribune, November 18, 2001

The Cleveland Clinic Men's Health Advisor, June 2002, page 3

Fumento, Michael, *The Fat of the Land Obesity Epidemic* (Viking Penguin Press), excerpted from The American Enterprise Institute for Public Policy Research, September 1997

Health, September 1999, page 23

Nutrition Action Newsletter, December 2001, page 3

Parenting, October 2001, page 111

Time, April 8, 2002, page 83

Wall Street Journal, May 1, 2000

CHAPTER 7

Ace Fitness Matters, May/June 2002, page 10

Conference of the American Society for Clinical Nutrition, February 26, 2002, San Diego, California, as reported in *Ace Fitness Matters,* May/June 2002, page 6

Consumer Reports on Health, June 2002

Fortune, February 18, 2002, page 36

Health, March 1999

The Heartland Health & Fitness Retreat, *The Heartland Cookbook,* Gillman, Illinois

McDonald's nutrition information pamphlet

Nutrition Action Newsletter, December 2001

Men's Health, April 2002, page 96

Parade, November 11, 2001, page 15

Self, August 2001, pages 125–27

Shape, May 2002, page 134

Tufts University Health & Nutrition Letter, June 2002, page 1

Wall Street Journal, May 1, 2000, page R4

CHAPTER 8

Ace Fitness Matters, March/April 2002, page 5

Fitness, April 2002

Good Housekeeping, November 1998, page 143

IDEA Health & Fitness Source, May 2001, page 35; September 2001, page 14; March 2002, page 11

New York Times, June 4, 2002, page F7

Newsweek, February 5, 2001, page 53

USA Today, July 12, 2001, page 9D

CHAPTER 9

IDEA Health & Fitness Source, September 2001, page 14; January 2002, page 10

New York Times, January 24, 2001, section 15, page 6

Nutrition Action Newsletter, January/February 2002, page 3; March 2002, page 8

O, The Oprah Magazine, April 2002

Parenting, December/January 2002, page 43; April 2002, page 38

Parents, March 2002, page 147

CHAPTER 10

Ace Fitness Matters, November/December 2001, page 5

Chicago Tribune, September 23, 2001, section 13, page 3

Health, May 1999, page 102

Mayo Clinic Health Letter, March 2002, page 4

Men's Health, April 2002

New York Times, June 24, 2001, section 15, page 6

Newsweek, Special Issue, Fall/Winter 2001, pages 36, 56

Rheumatic Diseases, February 2001

Town & Country

University of Texas Lifetime Health Letter, February 1992

USA Today, July 23, 2001, page 4D; February 27, 2002, page 5D

Wall Street Journal, May 1, 2002, page R5

CHAPTER 11

Shape, October 1999, page 24

Tufts University Heath & Nutrition Letter, January 2002

Index

About the Author

JIM KARAS, author of *The Business Plan for the Body* (Three Rivers Press), is a graduate of the Wharton School of Business and worked as a private portfolio manager before creating Jim Karas Personal Training, LLC (formerly Solo Sessions), the most successful weight-loss management firm in Chicago. A frequent guest on ABC's *Good Morning America* (he helped Diane Sawyer lose more than twenty-five pounds), he is also a contributing editor to *Good Housekeeping* magazine. He splits his time between New York and Chicago, where he lives with his wife and two children. Visit him at www.jimkaras.com.